The Mystery of the Dancing Plague: Unveiling the Science Behind Huntington's Disease

Navya

Table of contents

Introduction

1. Historical background

Since the Middle Ages, there have been oral and written reports describing "dancing disorders", what we now more commonly refer to as chorea (the Greek word for dance). Around the year 1000, involuntary, jerking and twitching movements were interpreted as consequences of curses and demonic possession (Vale and Cardoso, 2015). Hundreds of years later, this belief persisted and women persecuted during the witch hunt in Salem, Massachusetts, in the 1690s, were in fact affected by similar diseases (Vale and Cardoso, 2015). In the XIX century, the American physician George Huntington became interested in motor abnormalities and dementia in individuals of his community. He spent his life observing and collecting evidence in troubled middle-aged individuals who presented a family history of such disturbances. In 1872, his observations were published in *Medical and Surgical Reporter of Philadelphia* in manuscript entitled "On Chorea", where he described the disease that was later named after him (Huntington, 2003).

Further progress in the field of Huntington's disease (HD) would come during the HD Centenary Celebration in New York City, USA, when the work of the Venezuelan doctor Americo Negrette sparked the interest of the conference attendees. His report described an unusual cluster of HD-affected individuals in the geographically isolated village near the city of Maracaibo, Venezuela. Collecting testimonies from locals, he attempted to reconstruct the historical origin of HD and identify the patient zero, which he later confirmed as a European who had moved in the area in the 1860s (Bhattacharyya, 2016).

Under the leadership of the geneticist Nancy Wexler, a team of researchers travelled to Lake Maracaibo, intending to uncover the mutation that led to the development of HD. The study lasted 20 years during which blood samples and information on thousands of HD individuals were collected and shared globally between the members of the "Huntington's Disease Collaborative Research Group" (Wexler, 2012). Researchers and physicians were provided information for the identification of the causative gene. This extraordinary effort was brought by the Huntington's Disease Collaborative Research Group to achieve one of the most important milestones in the history of HD: the isolation of the mutation responsible for the disease (MacDonald et al., 1993).

2. Symptomatology

HD affects approximately 3 - 8 per 100,000 people worldwide, with a higher prevalence in western Europe, North America and Australia, where it reaches 5 - 13 people per 100,000 (Baig et al., 2016). HD is also known as Huntington's chorea, a definition that accurately describes its most characteristic motor features: spasms affecting the voluntary muscles (**Figure 1**). In adulthood, these involuntary movements occur in concomitance with other motor abnormalities such as dystonia, rigidity, akinesia and bradykinesia (Phillips et al., 2008). Notably, some HD patients, even prior to showing motor disturbances, display progressive cognitive impairments (Papp et al., 2011) that impact activities of daily living and that can progress into severe dementia (Peavy et al., 2010). Behavioral changes, such as mood disorders, depression, delusion, hallucinations and psychosis (**Figure 1**) commonly accompany the motor and cognitive features, troubling HD patients who, after 15 – 20 years, lose their autonomy and become bedbound. In the last years of the disease, death occurs due to heart failure (Abildtrup and Shattock, 2013) or aspiration pneumonia (Heemskerk and Roos, 2012). Notably, there is a wide variability of signs and symptoms within the HD population. Some gene carriers manifest mostly with motor disturbances and minimal mood or cognitive dysfunctions, while others suffer from cognitive and mood changes with limited motor symptoms (Hahn-Barma et al., 1998). Even though an inverse correlation exists between CAG repeat and the severity of symptoms, it does not fully explain the diversity of clinical profiles nor the progression patterns that are unique to each person (Andresen et al., 2007). A clear example of this is reported in a study in which monozygotic twins showed HD clinical phenotype 7 years apart, reinforcing the concept that disease onset is not exclusively determined by genetic factors (Friedman et al., 2005).

Although HD is a disease that mostly affects the central nervous system (CNS), it can also cause weight loss (Djoussé et al., 2002), skeletal muscle atrophy (Zielonka et al., 2014), testicular atrophy (Selvaraj et al., 2020) and cardiac problems that commonly lead to death (Abildtrup and Shattock, 2013).

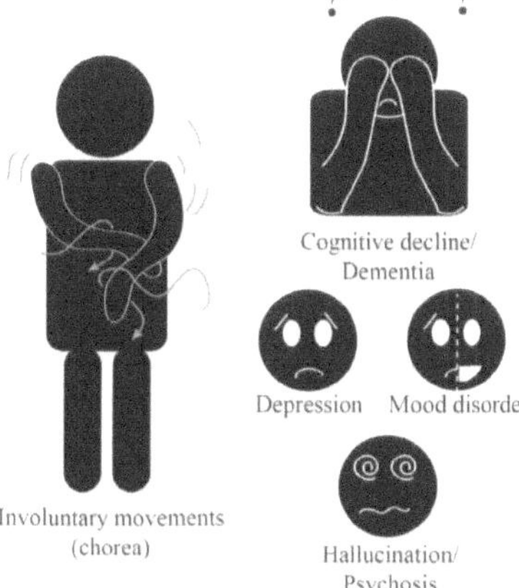

Figure 1. HD symptomatology. HD patients manifest with an array of motor, cognitive and psychiatric dysfunctions. Some of the most common motor symptoms consist of uncontrolled twerking movements defined as chorea. Cognitive symptoms, such as memory loss, learning difficulties, trouble in accomplishing the daily routine can degenerate into dementia. Psychiatric symptoms include depression, mood disorders, hallucinations and psychosis. Abbreviation: HD, Huntington's disease. Illustration made by Maria Masnata.

HD can also affect children (juvenile HD, JHD), who, in contrast to adults, do not always exhibit severe chorea or involuntary movements. Instead, juvenile cases are mainly affected by tremors and rigidity (Quarrell et al., 2013). Furthermore, a typical feature of JHD is the tendency to develop epileptic seizures, especially if the disease manifests before 10 years of age (Cloud et al., 2012; Gambardella et al., 2001). Similarly to adults, JHD individuals display cognitive impairments and behavioral changes, which can result in increased aggressiveness, apathy and poor scholastic performances (Ribaï et al., 2007). The progression of JHD is rather fast and the life expectancy does not exceed 10 to 15 years following the appearance of symptoms (Quarrell et al., 2013).

3. Neuropathology

The basal ganglia - a group of subcortical brain structures located deep in the brain - are the target of massive and progressive neurodegeneration in HD (Vonsattel et al., 1985). The basal ganglia span over two main brain subdivisions: the forebrain and the midbrain. The forebrain includes the dorsal striatum (caudate nucleus and putamen), the ventral striatum (nucleus accumbens and olfactory tubercle), the globus pallidus and the ventral pallidum. The substantia nigra and the diencephalon are found in the midbrain. Motor control and executive and cognitive functions are generated by these cerebral structures (Helie et al., 2013). In HD patients, the caudate nucleus and the putamen are the first structures affected by neurodegenerative processes (Vonsattel et al., 1985).

Within the striatum, the medium spiny neurons (MSNs) are the most vulnerable cellular elements. MSNs are GABAergic neurons, which give rise to two distinct pathways: the striatonigral (direct pathway) and the striatopallidal (indirect pathway) (Smith et al., 1998). The striatonigral pathway projects to the substantia nigra pars reticulata (SNr) or the internal segment of the globus pallidus (GPi) (Smith et al., 1998). The striatopallidal pathway projects to the external segment of the globus pallidus (GPe) (Gerfen, 1992). In the early stages of disease, the MSNs of the striatopallidal pathway, which also express dopaminergic D2 and enkephalin (ENK) receptors, are the first to degenerate (Crossman, 1987) (**Figure 2**). This is associated with the onset of involuntary movements (Crossman, 1987) (**Figure 2**). As the disease progresses, the MSNs of the striatonigral pathway, which express dopaminergic D1 receptors and substance P (SP), start dying and other motor dysfunction, such as rigidity and akinesia, begin to manifest (Berardelli et al., 1999) (**Figure 2**).

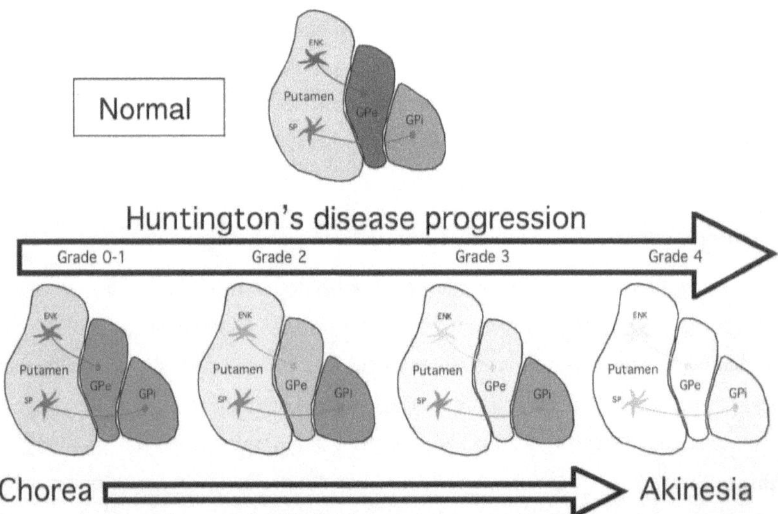

Figure 2. HD neuropathology. Schematic illustration of HD striatal degeneration according to Vonsattel grading scale and grade-relative motor symptoms. At grades 0 and 1, the striatum appears normal and

individuals mostly depict jerking and twitching movements (chorea). From grade 2 to 4, progressive loss of the ENK-GPe and SP-GPi projections is observed and is accompanied by progressive akinesia. At Grade 4, almost 95% of neurons have degenerated and the GPi, GPe and putamen are characterized by severe atrophy. Abbreviations: ENK, Enkephalin; GPe, External segment of the globus pallidus; GPi, Internal segment of the globus pallidus; SP, Substance P. Source (Reiner and Deng, 2018).

As HD progresses, other cerebral structures are affected by the neurodegenerative processes. For instance, the cortex is the second most affected forebrain structure (Cudkowicz and Kowall, 1990). More specifically, the large pyramidal cortical projection neurons, located in layers V and VI that project to the striatum, are the most vulnerable neuronal populations (Cudkowicz and Kowall, 1990; Hedreen et al., 1991). These neurons are part of the primary motor cortex, and their death arises in concomitance with motor impairments (Thu et al., 2010). Overtime, HD-associated neurodegeneration targets other areas such as the hippocampus (Begeti et al., 2016; Spargo et al., 1993; van den Bogaard et al., 2011). Neuronal death in the CA1 region (Spargo et al., 1993) and subsequent overall hippocampal atrophy (van den Bogaard et al., 2011) have been linked with the occurrence of cognitive impairments, in particular deficits in learning task (Begeti et al., 2016).

4. Genetics

Classified as an autosomal dominant neurodegenerative disease (**Figure 3A**), HD is caused by a mutation in the *HTT,* or *IT15,* gene. *HTT* is located on the short arm of chromosome 4 and codes for the protein huntingtin (HTT). The mutation consists of the insertion of more than 35 repetitions of the CAG trinucleotide in the exon 1 of the *HTT* gene (MacDonald et al., 1993) (**Figure 3B**). While 36 to 39 repeats are associated with reduced penetrance and an uncertain outcome, more than 40 CAG repeats result in HD onset (Myers, 2004). Moreover, the increase in the number of CAG repeats is a common feature during the transmission of genetic material (Maat-Kievit et al., 2001). Thus, if one of the parental chromosomes has 27 – 35 CAG repeats, a CAG expansion can occur, leading to HD-affected offspring (Maat-Kievit et al., 2001). The expanded (>35) CAG triplets encode a polyglutamine (polyQ) sequence in the mutant huntingtin protein (mHTT), which causes cytotoxicity that leads to neurodegeneration (Vonsattel and DiFiglia, 1998).

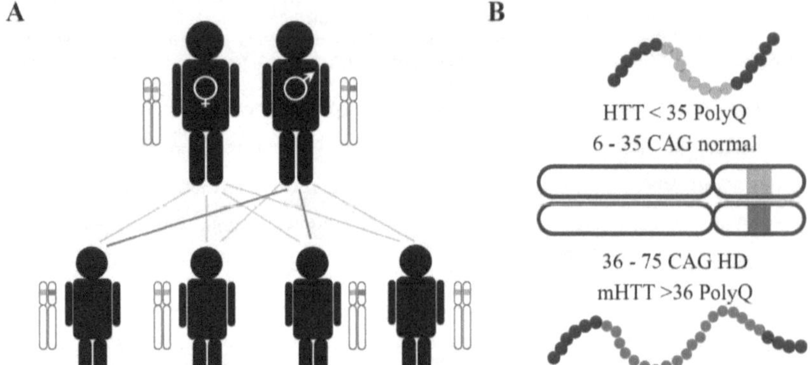

Figure 3. HD genetics. Schematic of the genetic transmission of the non-mutated (gray) and mutated (red) *HTT* gene (A) and of the chromosome 4 with non-mutated and mutated alleles and respective encoded proteins (B). The non-mutated *HTT* gene, with less than 36 CAG repeats, encodes for the HTT protein (< 35 polyQ), while the mutated *HTT* gene, with more than 36 CAG, encodes for mHTT (> 36 polyQ). Abbreviations: HD, Huntington's disease; HTT, Huntingtin; mHTT, Mutant huntingtin; PolyQ, polyglutamine. Illustration made by Maria Masnata.

5. Treatment

5.1 Pharmacological treatments

HD patients typically receive treatments to alleviate their symptoms, i.e. motor or mood disorders. To treat motor problems, more specifically involuntary movements (chorea), the drugs Tetrabenazine (Xenazine) and Deutetrabenazine (Austedo) are most often prescribed (Huntington Study Group, 2006; Yero and Rey, 2008). Tetrabenazine is well tolerated and ameliorates chorea when taken over extended periods of time (Fasano et al., 2008), however, it also causes a number of side-effects which include sedation, drowsiness, fatigue, insomnia, depression, suicidal thoughts, akathisia, anxiety and nausea (Huntington Study Group, 2006; Jankovic and Beach, 1997).

While selective serotonin reuptake inhibitors, such as citalopram (Celexa), fluoxetine (Prozac) and sertraline (Zoloft), are used to alleviate depression and are comparatively safe and efficient (De Marchi et al., 2001; Rowe et al., 2012), the treatment of psychosis is more challenging. Atypical antipsychotics, including risperidone (Risperdal), quetiapine (Seroquel) and olanzapine (Zyprexa), induce motor disturbances while typical antipsychotic, such as haloperidol (Haldol) and fluphenazine (Prolixin), suppress involuntary movements but in turn, can cause dystonia and rigidity (Unti et al., 2017).

At the moment, there are no available treatments to specifically improve cognition. Several candidates, approved by the Food and Drug Administration (FDA), have been tested in clinical trials, including Memantine (Beister et al., 2004; Cankurtaran et al., 2006) Lithium (Vestergaard et al., 1977) and Atomoxetine (Strattera) (Beglinger et al., 2009). However, none of these treatments have shown to significantly ameliorate cognitive deficits in HD (Beglinger et al., 2009; Beister et al., 2004; Cankurtaran et al., 2006).

The quest to find new symptomatic treatments, while exploring disease-modifying strategy, is still ongoing (Barker and Mason, 2019). For instance, a phase III clinical trial named PROOF-HD has just been launched (Teva Pharmaceutical Industry, 2016). This study investigates the drug Pridopidine (TV-7820), which is a dopamine stabilizer and an agonist of the sigma 1 receptor. It was initially thought to improve motor deficits in HD patients, but recent clinical trials reported just a trend towards amelioration of motor deficits (Prilenia, 2020), which was interpreted as sufficient evidence to pursue its evaluation.

5.2 Non-pharmacological treatments

5.2.1 Cell replacement therapy

Following the early success of cell transplantation in PD patients (Lindvall and Björklund, 2004), HD patients have also been considered candidates for cell replacement therapy. To this day, seven open-label trials were carried out to establish safety, tolerability and efficacy in this patient population. Trials were performed on a small number of patients with mild to advanced HD and yielded mild transient symptom improvements and a lack of long-term benefits (Bachoud-Lévi et al., 2000; Barker et al., 2013; Capetian et al., 2009; Gallina et al., 2010; Hauser et al., 2002; Kopyov et al., 1998; Maxan et al., 2018; Rosser et al., 2002). Post-mortem studies reported that the cellular grafts presented a progressive disease-like neuronal degeneration and an increase of microglial activation (Cicchetti et al., 2009; Maxan et al., 2018). Furthermore, mHTT aggregates, were detected within the neurons, infiltrating immune cells and extracellular matrix inside the boundaries of the grafted tissues (Cicchetti et al., 2014; Maxan et al., 2018). More recently, an open label study recruited a large cohort of patients (67 patients) to specifically evaluate the motor score between grafted and non-grafted patients (Assistance Publique - Hôpitaux de Paris, 2017). However, no motor improvements were reported, possibly due to graft rejection (alloimmunization). The authors suggested that the implantation of cell–derived neural precursors, instead of fetal human cells, could represent a better option to prevent graft rejection (Bachoud-Lévi and on behalf the Multicentric Intracerebral Grafting in Huntington's Disease Group, 2020).

5.2.2 Deep brain stimulation

Deep brain stimulation (DBS) is a treatment that consists of surgically implanting a device that delivers electrical signals to specific brain areas. This signal regulates the activity of the neuronal circuits responsible for motor abnormalities and can be controlled and modified according to the patients' needs. This technique was initially adopted to treat PD patients, showing significant improvement in motor symptoms (e.g. rigidity, tremors, bradykinesia, gait disturbances and problems with balance) (Deuschl et al., 2006; Williams et al., 2010). In HD patients, DBS of the internal segment of the globus pallidus has been proposed and tested on a small number of patients. Studies showed improvement of chorea, no effect on dystonia or cognition, but worsening of bradykinesia and rigidity (Delorme et al., 2016; Gonzalez et al., 2014; Velez-Lago et al., 2013; Wojtecki et al., 2015). Taken together, these results suggest that DBS could be beneficial for the treatment of chorea in HD patients, although long-term effects should be investigated.

5.3 Experimental treatments

5.3.1 Gene silencing and gene editing

Since HD is caused by a single genetic mutation, gene silencing and gene editing deserve serious consideration. Gene silencing through antisense oligonucleotide (ASO) consists of promoting mRNA degradation or blocking its translation, inducing a decrease in the synthesis of the target-protein. ASOs' potential for the treatment of HD was explored in preclinical trials with consistent reports of a high success rate in lowering mHTT and improving behavioral deficits in Hu97/18, an HD mouse model that fully expresses the human *HTT*, and YAC128 mice, an HD transgenic (Tg) mouse model overexpressing human full-length mHTT (Southwell et al., 2018; Stanek et al., 2013). Silencing of *HTT* with the

ASO drug IONIS-HTTRx is now under investigation in clinical trials (Tabrizi et al., 2019). IONIS-HTTRx is delivered intrathecally and aims to lower both normal HTT and mHTT in patients with early manifest HD. Results collected thus far show that ASO efficiently reduces mHTT CSF levels without serious side-effects (Mullard, 2019). However, treatment has not shown improvements in neurological outcomes, and no differences were observed between placebo-treated concerning cognitive and psychiatric symptoms or functional capacity (Smith and Tabrizi, 2019). IONIS-HTTRx is currently under investigation in the phase III trial "GENERATION HD1" (Hoffmann-La Roche, 2020).

While IONIS-HTTRx indiscriminately targets normal and mutated HTT, selective ASOs, such as WVE-120101 and WVE-120102, have now been trialed. This approach has been developed by WAVE Life and 2 trials are underway: PRECISION-HD1 recruited adult patients with early manifest HD who carry a targeted SNP rs362307 (SNP1), while PRECISION-HD2 was geared towards HD patients who carry an SNP rs362331 (SNP2) (Wave Life Sciences Ltd., 2020a, 2020b). The phase III reported reduced mHTT CSF levels by 12.4%, a much lower percentage in comparison to the one reported by IONIS-HTTRx, which reached 40 to 60% decrease in mHTT CSF content (Tabrizi et al., 2019). Higher doses are now being administered to the participants of the PRECISION-HD trials.

Preventing HTT synthesis by inhibiting translation could also be achieved using microRNAs. microRNAs are non-coding ribonucleic acid fragments that modulate gene expression. UniQure has developed the drug AMT-130, an adenoviral vector carrying a microRNA that non-selectively targets the HTT gene. As observed in the pre-clinical context, AMT-130 induced a dose-dependent HTT decrease and improvements in cognitive and anxiety-like behavior of Hu128/21 mice (Caron et al., 2020). The company has recently started testing AMT-130 in phase I and II clinical trials (UniQure Biopharma B.V., 2020).

The genome editing technique CRISPR/Cas9 was investigated in preclinical studies to address the pathological mutation of the *HTT* gene. CRISPR/Cas9 is a system of gene editing developed naturally by bacteria, which, in case of viral infections, can cut the viral DNA and prevent the virus from multiplying to attack the host. CRISPR/Cas9 has been tested and shown to inhibit the expression of mHTT aggregates in the striatum of KI140 mice, knock-in HD mice that contains 140 CAG repeats in the exon 1 of the *HTT* gene, successfully reducing the expression of mHTT and ultimately improving motor coordination and strength (Yang et al., 2017).

Gene silencing and gene editing are considered some of the most promising therapeutic approaches for the treatment of genetic disorders such as HD. For instance, in 2016, new ASO therapies were approved by the FDA for the treatment of the monogenic neuromuscular disorders Duchenne muscular dystrophy (DMD) and spinal muscular atrophy (SMA) (Commissioner, 2020a, 2020b). However, the long-term consequences and side effects of genome engineering are still unknown. It is therefore critical to investigate and closely monitor future clinical studies that target the *HTT* gene (Barker et al., 2020).

5.3.2 Immunotherapies

HD is characterized by abnormal hyper-activation of the immune system (Ciccocioppo et al., 2020). It has been established that the presence of pathogenic misfolded aggregates in the brain triggers a chronic immune response, mainly via activation of microglia, which in turn, release pro-inflammatory mediators including oxygen- and nitrogen-derived free radicals. This leads to progressive neuroinflammation, disruption of the integrity of the blood brain barrier and neuronal damage (Ciccocioppo et al., 2020; Sweeney et al., 2018). In the early stages of disease, reactive microglia have been detected in the neostriatum, cortex and globus pallidus, and their accumulation in the cortex and striatum directly linked to neuronal functionality and loss (Pavese et al., 2006; Sapp et al., 2001).

In recent years, several compounds have been identified as possible treatments to restore the physiological immune response in the brains of HD patients. Several of these drugs had been yielded promising results in animal studies and a selection went on to be tested in the clinic. Some of the drugs that reached phase II-III clinical trials are briefly discussed below:

- Pepinemab is an anti-SEMA4D monoclonal antibody developed by Vaccinex and the Huntington Study Group. Pepinemab's epitope is SEMA4D, a multifunctional transmembrane protein that regulates multiple neuroinflammation processes (Fisher et al., 2016). Intraperitoneal injections of the anti-SEMA4D antibody improved central and peripheral pathology as well as cognitive and anxiety-like behavior in YAC128 mice (Southwell et al., 2015). The inhibition of SEMA4D prevents astrogliosis, which would otherwise likely cause neuronal damage (Fisher et al., 2016; Southwell et al., 2015). Recently, Pepinemab was tested in the phase II SIGNAL clinical study, which recruited late prodromal or early manifest HD patients. Although the study did not fulfill the pre-established secondary outcomes (brain metabolic activity and behavioral improvements), a trend towards cognitive improvements, such as an amelioration in memory tasks and planning ability, was observed ("Top-line results of phase 2 SIGNAL study in Huntington's disease support potential for cognitive benefit of Pepinemab |Vaccinex, Inc.," n.d.). On the basis of these achievements, the FDA has conferred to Pepinemab the designation of "Orphan Drug" and "Fast Track" for the treatment of HD.

- Eicosapentaenoic acid (Ethyl-EPA) or Miraxion, a ω-3 fatty acid commonly used to treat hypertriglyceridemia, has been associated with anti-inflammatory properties. When administered to R6/1 mice - a transgenic model expressing exon 1 of the human *HTT* gene with approximately 114 CAG repeats - it significantly improved motor coordination and locomotor activity (Clifford et al., 2002), possibly by regulating the structure of the plasma membrane (Clifford et al., 2002), reducing oxidative stress (Puri et al., 2005) or inhibiting apoptosis (Murck and Manku, 2007). Ethyl-EPA was further investigated in the TREND-HD study by Amarin Neuroscience Ltd and the Huntington Study Group. It reached phase III, but failed to show clinical improvements, except for a small cohort of patients with a CAG repeat length shorter than 45 (Puri et al., 2005). After 12 months of treatment, these patients showed mild improvements on motor scores (Huntington Study Group TREND-HD Investigators, 2008). However, an additional clinical studiy detected no significant improvements in motor deficits in mild-to-moderate HD patients following 6 months of treatment with Ethyl-EPA (Ferreira et al., 2015).

- Laquinimod is an immunomodulator initially studied to treat multiple sclerosis. When tested in the R6/2 mouse model - a transgenic mouse which expresses exon 1 of the human *HTT* gene with approximately 125 CAG repeats - it reduced motor deficits and striatal pathology (Ellrichmann et al., 2017). Laquinimod's mechanism of action is unclear, but it seems to exert an anti-inflammatory action, reducing free radical damage (Ellrichmann et al., 2017). It is also thought to increase levels of brain-derived neurotrophic factor (BNDF), a pro-survival factor essential for the proper activity of the striatal neurons (Ellrichmann et al., 2017). The phase II trial for Laquinimod, named LEGATO-HD, was carried out by TEVA Pharmaceuticals for a total of 13 months. Ultimately, LEGATO-HD revealed that the compound did not meet the primary endpoints of the study, which consisted in the amelioration of baseline motor deficits (Teva Branded Pharmaceutical Products R&D, Inc., 2020).

Immunotherapies for HD have been explored since the early 2000s with inconsistent results between animal and human studies. For instance, minocycline, a tetracycline antibiotic, improved motor performances and extended life expectancy of R6/2 mice, seemingly by inhibiting apoptosis and decreasing oxidative stress and microglial activation (Chen et al., 2000; Tikka and Koistinaho, 2001). However, the absence of symptom improvements in mild to moderate functionally-impaired HD patients halted further clinical investigations (Huntington Study Group DOMINO Investigators, 2010). Modulating neuroinflammation is a challenging task, especially considering the complexity of its intricate pathways. Targeting specific elements, as does Pepinemab, could help avoid unwanted side effects and better predict overall results. Furthermore, immunotherapies could be excellent candidates in combinational therapies to tackle different neuropathological aspects of HD.

5.3.3 Antibody treatment

For several neurodegenerative disorders similar to HD, active (injection of antigens that would induce the organism's own immune response) or passive (injection of ready-made antibodies) immunization therapies have been tested in clinics with variable outcomes (Alpaugh and Cicchetti, 2019). For instance, while immunotherapies against Aβ have brought mixed results (Schilling et al., 2018), tau immunotherapies are now gaining momentum (Congdon and Sigurdsson, 2018). Either anti-tau active or passive immunization has been demonstrated to be safe and to significantly improve AD pathology and cognitive deficit (Congdon and Sigurdsson, 2018). For HD, antibody-based therapies are still in early stage of development and no compounds have yet been translated to the clinic.

Active immunization against mHTT has been evaluated by injections of plasmids containing mHTT N-terminal fragment with 103 polyQ administered to R6/2 mice (Miller et al., 2003). Treated animals promptly developed an immune response against the antigen and, despite no effect being detected with respect to the number of mHTT aggregates, the treatment improved the diabetic phenotype of these mice (Miller et al., 2003). Other studies have tested antibodies (passive immunization) which target extracellular mHTT, i.e. the caspase-6 cleaved mHTT fragments enzyme (aa586)) (Bartl et al., 2020). This antibody, developed by AFFiRiS and referenced to as mAB C6-17, efficiently prevented cell-to-cell mHTT propagation in *in vitro* systems, decreasing by more than 90% the uptake of HTTExon1Q103 by healthy acceptor cells (Bartl et al., 2020). Antibodies directed against intracellular mHTT (intrabodies) have also been developed (Amaro and Henderson, 2016). For example INT41, which specifically targets proline-rich region of HTT, was administered to R6/2 mice using a recombinant AAV and shown to induce a reduction of mHTT aggregates within the striatum (Amaro and Henderson, 2016).

Research in the field of immunotherapy has made significant progress in the development of treatments for AD and PD (Alpaugh and Cicchetti, 2019), and is now being considered for HD (Denis et al., 2019). Antibody-based therapies have the distinct advantage of being highly specific to the selected epitopes and can target intracellular or extracellular mHTT both in the periphery and CNS. The antibodies' low molecular weight makes them suitable for nanocarrier-based delivery approaches to control the rate of antibody release, reduce antibody degradation and prevent unwanted host immune response (Wagh and Law, 2013). Based on the concept that mHTT is frequently found outside the cell boundary (Cicchetti et al., 2014; Drouin-Ouellet et al., 2015; Tan et al., 2015; Wild et al., 2015), active and passive immunization strategies targeting extracellular mHTT are attracting interest (Denis et al., 2019).

6. HD animal models

Animal models allow the study of pathophysiological and behavioral changes in disease-engineered living organisms and they represent one of the most powerful resources to study novel therapeutic strategies. The development of more relevant models of HD followed the discovery of the *HTT* gene mutation, with the elaboration of transgenic mouse models that expressed exon 1 of the human *HTT* gene, known as the R6 line (Mangiarini et al., 1996). Four R6 mice were generated, two of which, the R6/1 and R6/2, are still commonly used in HD research for their disease-like phenotype. The two models slightly differ in terms of their behavioral and neuropathological characteristics (Mangiarini et al., 1996). The R6/1 mice express 114 CAG repeats, develop a motor behavior at 15–21 weeks of age, and mHTT aggregates at 2 months of age (**Table 1**). On the other hand, the R6/2 model is notorious for developing an early-onset HD phenotype (**Table 1**). R6/2 mice express 144 to 150 CAG repeats and show the first signs of motor and cognitive deficits starting from 3 weeks of age. The appearance of intranuclear mHTT aggregates begins soon after birth and proceeds aggressively (Mangiarini et al., 1996).

Shortly after the arrival of the R6 mice, another transgenic mouse model was developed which, in contrast to the R6, expresses the full-length human *HTT* (Hodgson et al., 1999). It was generated using a yeast artificial chromosome (YAC) containing a full-length human *HTT* with expanded polyQ repeats (Hodgson et al., 1999) (**Table 1**). The YAC128 mice depict motor deficits at 4 months of age (Menalled et al., 2009) and cognitive deficits at 8 months of age (Van Raamsdonk et al., 2005). Accumulation of nuclear mHTT aggregates starting from 6 months of age is associated with decreased striatal volume and selective striatal neurodegeneration (Hodgson et al., 1999; Slow et al., 2003). As the YAC128, the BACHD model was generated using a bacterial artificial chromosome (BAC), expressing the human full-length human *HTT* gene (**Table 1**). BACHD mice are characterized by progressive motor impairments starting at 2 months of age (Menalled et al., 2009), while mHTT aggregates are detected after 6 months of age (Gray et al., 2008).

Chimeric knock-in (KI) models, expressing the human exon 1 of the *HTT* gene with CAG expansion, were also engineered to model HD. The KI140 mouse was designed by inserting the human *HTT* exon 1, with approximately 120-140 CAG repeats, into the mouse *Htt* (Menalled et al., 2003) (**Table 1**). The mice manifest complex motor deficits, with initial hyperactivity at 1 month of age followed by a progressive decrease in locomotor activity starting from 4 weeks (Menalled et al., 2009). Numerous mHTT aggregates, predominantly in the striatum and cortex, are detectable starting from 4 months of age (Menalled et al., 2003) (**Table 1**). The zQ175 mouse model, which originates from the KI140, expresses the human *HTT* exon1 with 188 CAG repeats and slightly differs in behavioral phenotype. It displays motor and learning deficits starting at 6 months of age (Menalled et al., 2012). It additionally develop an age-dependent accumulation of mHTT aggregates mostly in the striatum and cortex. Nuclear mHTT inclusions are visible in the striatum (4 months of age) and in cortex (8 months of age) (Menalled et al., 2012).

Model	Genetic manipulation	Behavioral Changes	Neuropathology	References
R6/1	Expression of exon 1 of the human *HTT* gene containing 116 CAG	Motor performance abnormalities at 15–21 weeks of age Body weight loss Comparatively short live span (32–40 weeks)	Reduced brain volume by 18 weeks of age Neuronal atrophy in absence of overall neuronal loss Deposition of mHTT aggregates starting from 2 months of age	(Mangiarini et al., 1996)
R6/2	Expression of exon 1 of the human *HTT* gene containing 144-150 CAG	Motor symptoms starting from 4-6 weeks of age (clasping, loss of motor coordination, stereotypic involuntary movements, shaking, reduced locomotor activity) Cognitive symptoms from (impaired short and long-term and working memory; early-onset learning deficit) Anxiety-like behavior (tendency to stay in the dark) Epileptic seizure Body weight loss Short live span (12 – 18 weeks)	Reduced brain volume, particularly of the striatum Progressive neuronal atrophy with neuronal loss at 12 weeks of age Extended mHTT aggregates deposition staring at day 1 post-birth	(Carter et al., 1999; Mangiarini et al., 1996; Menalled et al., 2009)
YAC128	Expression of the human *HTT* with 128 CAG repeats	Motor deficit (loss of motor coordination; initially mild hypoactive then hypokinetic) Weight gain	Accumulation of nuclear mHTT aggregates starting from 6 months of age Decreased brain weight and striatal volume starting from 12 months of age	(Hodgson et al., 1999; Menalled et al., 2009; Slow et al., 2005, 2003)
BACHD mice	Expression of the human *HTT* with 97–98 CAG repeats	Motor deficit (loss of motor coordination at 4 weeks of age; hypoactivity) Anxiety-like behavior (higher preference for the dark)	Brain atrophy starting from 12 months (loss of cortical and striatal volume) Diffuse nuclear accumulation of mHTT aggregates starting from 6 months of age	(Gray et al., 2008; Menalled et al., 2009)

		Weight gain	Higher frequency of aggregates in the cortex than in the striatum	
KI140	Insertion of *HTT* exon 1 (with ≅ 120-140 CAG repeats) into the mouse *Htt*	Motor deficits (initial hyperactivity followed by a progressive hypoactivity; gait abnormalities) Body weight loss	Presence of mHTT aggregates predominantly in the striatum and cortex at 4 months of age Abnormal neuronal activity	(Menalled et al., 2009; Miller et al., 2011)
zQ175	Insertion of *HTT* exon 1 (with ≅ 120-188 CAG repeats) into the mouse *Htt*	Motor deficits (hyperactivity; motor incoordination; gait abnormalities) Cognitive deficit (learning deficit) Body weight loss	Age-dependent accumulation of mHTT aggregates mostly in the striatum and cortex Nuclear mHTT inclusions appear first in the striatum (4 months of age) and after in the cortex (8 months of age) Decreased levels of Drd2; DARPP32; GLT1	(Carty et al., 2015; Menalled et al., 2012)

Table 1. Most commonly used HD mouse models. Abbreviations: DARPP32, Dopamine- and cAMP-regulated neuronal phosphoprotein; Drd2, Dopamine receptor D2; GLT1, Glutamate transporter 1; HTT, Huntingtin; mHTT, Mutant huntingtin. Table made by Maria Masnata.

7. HD, a proteinopathy

HD, as Alzheimer's disease (AD) and Parkinson's disease (PD), belongs to the family of neurodegenerative diseases defined as proteinopathy. Proteinopathies are caused by proteins that adopt an abnormal structural configuration, assemble into progressively more complex structures and eventually form insoluble aggregates (Soto and Pritzkow, 2018). This process induces cellular damage and ultimately cell death. Each proteinopathy is associated with one or more proteins that actively contribute to neuropathological changes. For instance in AD, amyloid precursor protein (APP) as well as tau misfold and aggregate respectively into senile plaques and neurofibrillary tangles (NFTs) or neuropil threads (NTs) (Serrano-Pozo et al., 2011). In PD, the distinctive histopathological signatures are Lewy bodies (LBs), aggregates mostly composed of the protein α-synuclein (α-syn) (Spillantini et al., 1998). In HD, the acknowledged player in neurodegeneration is mHTT, whose polyQ expansion induces abnormal protein folding and aggregation which confer a toxic gain of function to the protein (DiFiglia et al., 1997). The aggregation process and putative gain of function mechanisms of mHTT will be discussed in detail in the following paragraphs (section 9).

Recently a growing body of evidence has further indicated that mHTT may not be the sole protein involved in HD and that tau could also contribute to pathology at both genetic and molecular levels (Gratuze et al., 2016). At the genetic level, although no tau (*MAPT*) mutations have yet been reported in HD patients (Moss et al., 2017), individuals with H2 *MAPT* haplotype manifest with a more severe cognitive decline (Vuono et al., 2015). Furthermore, altered exon 10 splicing of *MAPT* has been identified in HD patients, resulting in an increased expression of 4R tau isoforms (Fernández-Nogales et al., 2014). Because of its increased concentration, 4R tau was detected into nuclear rod structures within the striatum of HD patients (Fernández-Nogales et al., 2014). At the histopathological levels, increased levels of soluble and insoluble hyperphosphorylated tau (NFTs and NTs), mainly in the putamen and cortex, (Caparros-Lefebvre et al., 2009; Davis et al., 2014; St-Amour et al., 2018; Vuono et al., 2015) can be observed. Taken together, emerging evidence suggests that tau might take part in HD neurodegenerative processes.

8. The Huntingtin protein

HTT is a large (350 kDa) protein encoded by the *HTT* gene. The *HTT* gene is widely expressed among metazoans, thus highly conserved among vertebrates (Baxendale et al., 1995; Li et al., 1999; Tartari et al., 2008). In higher vertebrates, HTT is expressed in embryos and is essential for survival, since the depletion of the *HTT* mouse homolog ($Hdh^{-/-}$) induces embryonic death (Duyao et al., 1995; Nasir et al., 1995; Zeitlin et al., 1995). In humans, HTT is highly expressed in the brain, testes, cardiovascular system, skeleton and digestive tract (Strong et al., 1993). In the brain, HTT is expressed by both neurons and glial cells (Landwehrmeyer et al., 1995). Within neurons, HTT is frequently found associated with other proteins in the nucleus as well as in the cytoplasm, bound to the cytoplasmic membrane, organelles or vesicles (Saudou and Humbert, 2016). HTT is involved in several physiological functions, such as transcriptional regulation, axonal trafficking, endocytosis and cellular death (DiFiglia et al., 1995). The following paragraphs describe the currently known HTT functions and how mHTT may interfere with them.

- <u>Transcription.</u> Transcription, the copy of genetic information from DNA to RNA, is the first of the two key elements of gene expression. This is followed by translation, the transfer of genetic information from RNA to proteins (Kornberg, 2007). HTT, as a transcriptional regulator, is responsible for the conversion of DNA to mRNA (Saudou and Humbert, 2016). In particular, WT HTT binds to numerous transcription factors that are involved in the transcription of hormones (Steffan et al., 2000), tumor suppression (Steffan et al., 2000) and inflammation agents (Takano and Gusella, 2002). On the other hand, mHTT can sequester transcriptional regulators and impair the transcription of various proteins, such as the BDNF. For example, in the cortex of YAC72 mice, mHTT expression is associated with reduced BDNF production, which results in neuronal death (Zuccato et al., 2001).

- Axonal transport. Axonal transport is a cellular mechanism responsible for the movement of organelles, such as mitochondria or synaptic vesicles, or molecules, including lipids and proteins, from the soma towards the synaptic terminal (anterograde transport) (Maday et al., 2014). This process also helps molecules to be transported from the axon to the soma, where they can be digested (retrograde transport) (Maday et al., 2014). HTT is an essential component of the machinery involved in axonal transport, where it acts as a regulatory factor for vesicular transport. HTT binds to Huntingtin-associated protein 1 (HAP1), which mediates HTT interactions with kinesin (anterograde transport) and with dynein and its cofactor dynactin (retrograde transport) (Block-Galarza et al., 1997). HTT facilitates the axonal transport of vesicles containing various proteins and receptors, including BDNF, autophagosomes, endosomes and lysosomes (Caviston and Holzbaur, 2009; Gauthier et al., 2004; Saudou and Humbert, 2016). In cultured striatal neurons transfected with the HTTExon1Q120, mHTT has been shown to accumulate within axonal projections, hindering the axonal transport (Li et al., 2001).

- Endocytosis. Endocytosis is a cellular mechanism that controls various cellular functions such as internalization and recycling of plasma membrane components/ligands as well as the uptake and degradation of macromolecules and extracellular particles. HTT regulates endocytic pathways, including the clathrin-mediated endocytosis (Metzler et al., 2001) and the endosomal trafficking (Pal et al., 2006). In the immortalized striatal neuronal progenitors expressing Q111 (STHdhQ111/Q111), mHTT interferes with endocytic processes, perturbing cellular homeostasis and consequently inducing accumulation of intracellular cholesterol and relocation of membrane proteins (Borgonovo et al., 2013; Trushina et al., 2006).

- <u>Autophagy.</u> Autophagy, the cellular machinery responsible to degrade protein and organelles, is governed by several proteins including HTT, which, in turn, regulates autophagy through numerous and complementary mechanisms. For instance, HTT is involved in the axonal transport of autophagosomes (Wong and Holzbaur, 2014) and binds p62, an autophagy receptor, to control autophagy (Rui et al., 2015). While the expansion of the polyQ stretch in mHTT compromises the normal autophagy functioning (Martin et al., 2015), reducing mHTT promotes autophagy and increases the longevity of KI140 HD mice (Zheng et al., 2010).

- <u>Apoptosis.</u> Programmed cell death is a multistep process, which is modulated by an enzymatic reaction involving caspases. HTT promotes cell survival by inhibiting the activation of the pro-apoptotic enzymes caspase-3 and -9 (Rigamonti et al., 2000) In contrast, the expression of truncated mHTT with expanded polyQ (Q60 and Q150), as tested in N2A cells, is linked to increased activation of caspases-1, -3 and -9 (Chen et al., 2000; Jana et al., 2001; Ona et al., 1999). Notably, inhibiting caspase-1, -3 and -9 in the CNS extends the life span of R6/2 mice (Chen et al., 2000).

9. The mutant huntingtin protein

As a result of the CAG expansion in the *HTT* gene, mHTT presents an elongated polyQ stretch at the N-terminal region (Sieradzan et al., 1999). As WT HTT, mHTT is also ubiquitously expressed and both proteins share similarities and differences in intracellular location, activity and degradation processes (Strong et al., 1993). While WT HTT is predominantly observed in the axons, mHTT is more often detected in the cell bodies (Gourfinkel-An et al., 1997). In particular, mHTT is observed in the soma of striatal, cortical and thalamic neurons and its concentration correlates with the length of the CAG repeat expansion (Gourfinkel-An et al., 1997).

The elongated polyQ stretch at the N-terminus of the mHTT protein confers the propensity to misfold and aggregate (Sieradzan et al., 1999). Several models have been developed to explain the aggregation process. One of them is the "multistep aggregation model", which suggests that mHTT aggregation occurs in consecutive steps (Ossato et al., 2010). Another widely accredited model sustains that mHTT aggregation is a dynamic process, where small and large species of mHTT assemble and disassemble concurrently (Legleiter et al., 2010; Soto and Pritzkow, 2018) (**Figure 4**).

This multistep aggregation process is divided into 4 main phases: in phase 1, soluble misfolded monomers accumulate; in phase 2, soluble misfolded monomers give rise to the formation of small oligomers; in phase 3, the increasing load of structurally abnormal monomers and oligomers triggers the nucleation stage and in phase 4, the nucleation stage concludes with the formation of insoluble inclusion bodies (IBs) (Ossato et al., 2010) (**Figure 4A**). Importantly at this final stage, WT HTT is recruited into the IBs through its N-terminus (Ossato et al., 2010), contributing to the depletion of WT HTT and compromising the roles of HTT (HTT loss of function) (Rajan et al., 2001).

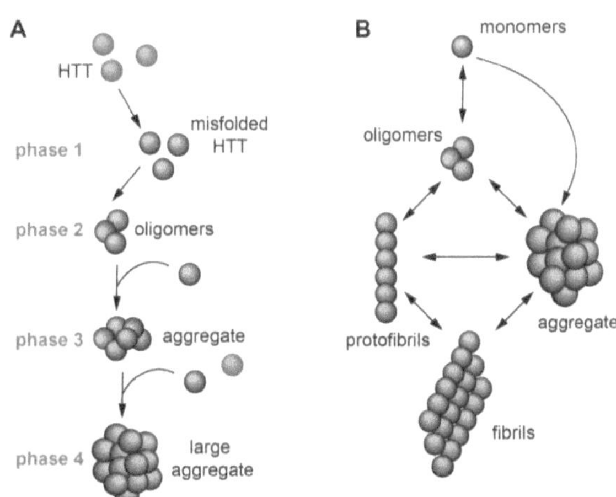

Figure 4. mHTT aggregation models. On the left (**A**), the multistep aggregation model indicates that more complex species are formed starting at phase 1 until the formation of a large insoluble aggregate in phase 4. The interchanging and dynamic formation of different mHTT species is illustrated on the right (**B**). Abbreviation: HTT, huntingtin. Illustration made by Maria Masnata.

In contrast to the multistep model, other studies suggest that the aggregation process is not a linear sequence of events, but a dynamic series of conformational changes and protein bindings that occur in parallel, or simultaneously (Legleiter et al., 2010; Soto and Pritzkow, 2018) (**Figure 4B**). Oligomers, in particular, are the most dynamic species and they are in equilibrium with smaller mHTT forms, such as monomers, or with more complex ones, such as fibrils. Furthermore, oligomers are capable of permanently aggregating into IBs (Soto and Pritzkow, 2018). Notably, all studies agree that the aggregation process depends on the polyQ length; the longer the polyQ strain, the quicker the aggregation process (Arrasate et al., 2004; Drombosky et al., 2018; Legleiter et al., 2010).

Another debated issue is the identification of the mHTT pathogenic entity among large aggregates, soluble oligomers, fibrils and soluble monomers (Ast et al., 2018; Caughey and Lansbury, 2003; DiFiglia et al., 1997; Pieri et al., 2012; Scherzinger et al., 1997) (**Figure 5**). Initially, the end-products of mHTT aggregation – the large insoluble IBs – were considered the main culprits in neuronal death (Davies et al., 1997; DiFiglia et al., 1997). This hypothesis was based on post-mortem observations of R6/2 mice brains which revealed that the deposition of nuclear IBs, similar to those identified in HD brains, appeared in concomitance with behavioral deficits (Davies et al., 1997; DiFiglia et al., 1997). However, *in vitro* models in which mHTT expression is induced by adenoviral (Dong et al., 2012) or lentiviral vectors (Zala et al., 2005), have revealed that cortical neurons accumulate a significant number of

IBs, but with no clear toxic consequences. In contrast, striatal neurons develop significant morphological changes that are accompanied by the loss of neurofilaments and ultimately cell death, despite the fact that mHTT aggregates are rarely seen within these cells (Dong et al., 2012; Zala et al., 2005). In agreement with these findings, post-mortem human tissue shows elevated concentration of IBs in the cortex rather than in the striatum, suggesting that IBs localization and density does not associate with cell death (Gutekunst et al., 1999).

Some studies have suggested that large aggregates can be protective, while soluble mHTT was instead to be blamed for cytotoxicity (Arrasate et al., 2004; Arrasate and Finkbeiner, 2012). This hypothesis was supported by *in vitro* work using primary culture of rat striatal neurons transfected with N-terminal fragment of HTTExon1Q72 or Q103, where it was observed that the neurons with larger IBs survived longer than neurons with smaller mHTT aggregates (Arrasate et al., 2004). Several other *in vitro* experiments confirmed that cell survival was independent of IBs, but correlated with the presence of soluble mHTT (Lajoie and Snapp, 2010; Takahashi et al., 2008). Furthermore, in mice expressing the human mHTT N-truncated form, the widespread deposition of mHTT aggregates does not associate with behavioral changes (Slow et al., 2005), while in mice expressing the full-length human mHTT, motor and cognitive deficits occur despite scarce mHTT aggregates (Slow et al., 2005). Collectively, *in vitro* and *in vivo* evidence indicates that IBs are unrelated to pathological outcomes, and could instead signify a coping response to pathogenic stressors (Arrasate and Finkbeiner, 2012).

Unlike IBs, mHTT soluble oligomers are currently considered culprits of HD cytotoxicity (Saudou et al., 1998; Takahashi et al., 2008). However, determining how oligomers induce cytotoxicity is particularly challenging due to their propensity to rapidly shift conformation and form larger aggregates or disaggregate into monomers. Some fluorescence microscopy techniques have proven useful to study the process of oligomer formation. For instance, they provided evidence that, in living cells, mHTT oligomers induce a higher death rate than insoluble mHTT aggregates (Herrera et al., 2011; Lajoie and Snapp, 2010; Takahashi et al., 2008) and could be used as a tool to test novel therapeutic approaches to tackle toxic derivates of the mHTT aggregation process (He et al., 2020). Although the cytotoxicity of oligomers has been demonstrated, a study that performed a direct comparison between syntenic oligomers and fibrils showed that fibrils alone, binding the plasma membrane and disrupting Ca^{2+} levels, induced apoptosis in cultured murine and human neuron-like cells (N2A and SH-SY5Y) (Monsellier et al., 2016; Pieri et al., 2012; Trevino et al., 2012). Furthermore, a variety of studies on mammalian cell lines (Cos-7, HEK, N2A, CHO, HeLa) exposed to synthetic fibrils of exon 1 of HTT with an expanded polyQ stretch reported that these fibrils were readily taken up by all of these cell lines. Once taken up, fibrils acted as 'seeds', recruiting endogenous soluble HTT into larger aggregates (Ren et al., 2009; Trevino 2012; Ruiz-Arlandis et al., 2016) (**Figure 5**). A recent work comparing fibrils with small soluble mHTT monomers suggested that mHTT exon1 monomers induced a higher seeding activity *in vitro* (Ast et al., 2018). Seeding-competent mHTT exon1 monomers were further detected in the brains of pre-symptomatic R6/2 mice and were increasingly more abundant with disease progression (Ast et al., 2018), supporting their contribution to HD pathology. The concept of protein propagation and seeding will be further discussed in sections 10-12.

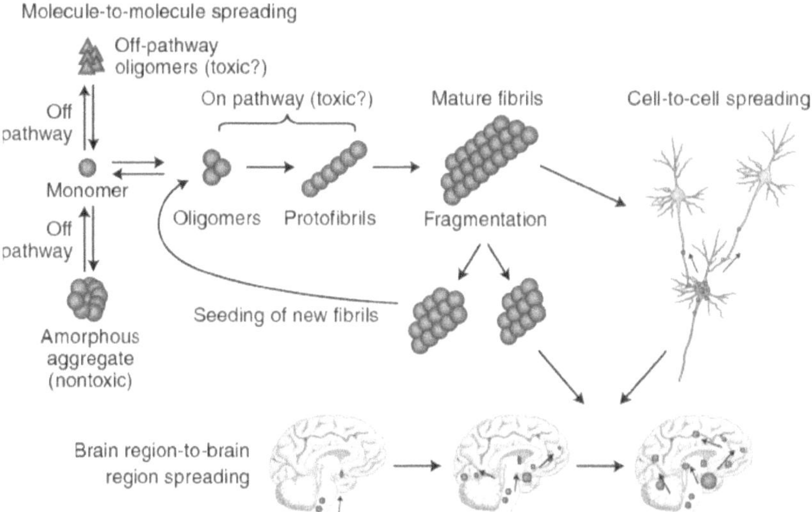

Figure 5. Protein aggregation and the prion-like propagation. Protein monomers can misfold and assemble in progressively larger structures such oligomers and fibrils. Those toxic protein forms can further recruit smaller species into new fibrils, amplifying the aggregation process. The newly formed protein entities can propagate between cells and across different brain regions spreading pathology. Source (Soto and Pritzkow, 2018).

Also of importance is the fact that the pathogenicity of mHTT seems to be associated to both on a gain and a loss of function of the normal HTT protein. mHTT displays new functions conferred by the polyQ expansion, which trigger the protein to misfold and aggregate in progressively more complex structures (DiFiglia et al., 1997). However, and as previously mentioned, not all sub-products of mHTT aggregations are linked to neuronal death; some of them may be considered coping responses of an underlying toxic process (Arrasate et al., 2004). Thus, the hypothesis that the loss of function may contribute to HD development is gaining consent. To verify this theory, mice models have been genetically engineered to express different HTT levels. The total inactivation of the mouse *Hdh* gene causes early embryonic lethality, indicating that HTT is essential for proper neurodevelopment (Duyao et al., 1995; Nasir et al., 1995; Zeitlin et al., 1995). In contrast, silencing *Hdh* in the mouse forebrain during embryogenesis or early post-natally is not lethal, but it does induce a behavioral and physiological HD-like phenotype (Dragatsis et al., 2000). Motor deficits, reduced life span and neuronal loss in the striatum and cortex have been detected in animals lacking HTT within the forebrain, suggesting the importance of HTT in neurodevelopment (Dragatsis et al., 2000). These findings are supported by a number of *in vivo* and *in vitro* studies, which demonstrate that in the presence of mHTT, HTT functions (transcriptional regulation, axonal transport, endocytosis, autophagy and apoptosis) are impaired (Borgonovo et al., 2013; Li et al., 2001; Martin et al., 2015; Trushina et al., 2006; Zheng et al., 2010; Zuccato et al., 2001).

10. Prions and prion-like proteins

In the 1900s, the attention of the scientific community was drawn to a disease affecting sheep and goats in the United Kingdom and which was characterized by abnormal behavior followed by death. This disease was termed *scrapie* and was extremely feared by farmers, as it was considered highly infectious and incurable. In the late XX century, the scientist Stanley Prusiner investigated the phenomenon and identified the structure of the agent responsible for scrapie (Prusiner, 1982). He observed that this agent possessed unique biological properties that differentiated it from viruses, plasmids and viroids, in part by its sensitivity to proteases and resistance to nucleic acid degradation (Prusiner, 1982). He described this new entity as "prion", which stands for "proteinaceous infectious particles" (Prusiner, 1982).

While human diseases caused by prion, such as Creutzfeldt-Jakob disease (CJD), are extremely rare, recent studies have demonstrated that pathological proteins responsible for much more common neurodegenerative disorders seem to behave in a prion-like fashion (Prusiner, 2012) (**Figure 5**). Indeed, the discovery of Lewy-body pathology within fetal ventral mesencephalic cells grafted in patients with PD years earlier has radically changed our views on the potential pathogenic mechanisms underlying sporadic neurodegenerative disorders of the CNS. This observation, initially reported by two independent teams (Kordower et al., 2008; Li et al., 2008), has led to the theory that the pathogenic α-syn protein can spread from the diseased brain to healthy tissue and cause protein aggregation and cellular dysfunction in a prion-like fashion (Brundin et al., 2010; Olanow and Prusiner, 2009; Soto, 2012). Accordingly, it has been demonstrated both *in vitro* and *in vivo* that α-syn, the main component of Lewy bodies, can be released into the extracellular space and then be internalized by neighboring neurons (Desplats et al., 2009; Hansen et al., 2011), acting as a toxic agent that could seed pathology in the process. Furthermore, intracerebral inoculation of brain homogenates derived from aged α-syn transgenic mice, or injections of synthetic α-syn preformed fibrils, accelerates the formation of protein aggregates and precipitates neurological dysfunction in small animals (Luk et al., 2012a, 2012b). It is also now known that there is pathology remote from the injection sites in these types of studies, which further supports an intercellular transneuronal spread of protein, as has also been demonstrated in rodent allografts placed in animals expressing human α-syn (Angot et al., 2012). In the latter study, human α-syn was shown to colocalize with markers of endosomes and exosomes (Angot et al., 2012), which could represent one of the routes by which the protein is transferred (Angot et al., 2012; Goedert et al., 2010). This mode of protein spread and disease propagation has been shown experimentally with several other proteins including amyloid and tau (Guo and Lee, 2014; Jucker and Walker, 2013; Soto, 2012). However, these studies have proposed a number of other putative mechanisms for protein spread which include nanotubes (Saida Abounit et al., 2016; Costanzo et al., 2013), vesicular transport (Angot et al., 2012; Lee et al., 2012), endocytosis (Hansen et al., 2011; Ruiz-Arlandis et al., 2016; Wu et al., 2013) or even direct penetration of the plasma membrane (Ren et al., 2009) (**Figure 6**).

What is emerging from all this work is that a number of these processes may be common to all neurodegenerative disorders, not just sporadic but also monogenic diseases such as HD (Brundin et al., 2010; Cicchetti et al., 2014; Soto, 2012). In HD, recent evidence has added weight to the idea that mHTT – the genetic product that defines the disease – can propagate from cell-to-cell. *In vivo* observations for the ability of mHTT to travel across synapses has been collected in embryonic human stem cells differentiated into neurons and implanted in R6/2 mice (Pecho-Vrieseling et al., 2014). It has also been demonstrated by expressing the human *HTT* gene (138 CAG) within olfactory receptor neurons which was subsequently found in the synaptically connected large posterior neurons in the brain of drosophila (Babcock and Ganetzky, 2015). Various cell types (HEK), including neuron-like cells (Cos-7 and PC-12), have been shown to internalize synthetic mHTT aggregates from the extracellular milieu (Ren et al., 2009; Yang et al., 2002). The aggregates can be either translocated to the nucleus where their pathogenic effects on transcription can be exerted, leading to cell dysfunction and death, (Yang et al., 2002) or act as seeds for further protein aggregation within the cell itself (Herrera et al., 2011). Prion-like spread has also been suggested to take place following the phagocytosis of mHTT aggregates by glial cells in a *Drosophila* model of HD. The engulfed aggregates gained access to the cytoplasm of microglia where they interacted with soluble HTT, initiating a prion-like dissemination of pathology (Pearce et al., 2015). Since mHTT were detected into infiltrating CD8+ immune cells (Maxan et al., 2018), this is a likely scenario that may, at least partly, contribute to HD pathology and that certainly cannot be ruled out at this stage.

11. Evidence for mHTT prion-like behavior *in vitro* and putative spreading mechanisms

11.1 Transneuronal/transsynaptic propagation

The transsynaptic propagation theory (**Figure 6**) has gained additional support with the work of Pecho-Vrieseling et al. (Pecho-Vrieseling et al., 2014). In this study, the authors generated mixed-genotype (R6/2-wild-type (WT)) cortico-striatal cultures, more specifically combining R6/2 striatal neurons with WT cortical neurons or WT striatal neurons with R6/2 cortical neurons. Functional R6/2 cortical-WT striatal networks were created and used to study long-distance mHTT propagation from the cortex to WT DARPP-32+ MSN. However, this was not seen in the R6/2 striatum-WT cortical circuit, as no significant amounts of mHTT aggregates were detected in the WT cortex.

In a second set of experiments, the authors used embryonic human stem cells differentiated into neurons and tagged with GFP (hGFP) which they then transplanted into organotypic brain slices derived from R6/2 mice. Cell inoculations were performed within the cortex and striatum and the identity of the transplanted cells was confirmed by immunostainings of mature and structure-specific cellular markers such as Tbr1 (cortex) and DARPP-32 (striatum). Two waves of mHTT accumulation were seen between the mouse neurons: one wave occurred at 3–4 weeks and a second took place between 6–8 weeks following the initiation of cultures. In the human transplanted cells, mHTT accumulation progressively increased within the striatum between 4 and 8 weeks at which point it plateaued, while in the cortex, the pattern of propagation was identical to that seen in mouse neurons. The impact of mHTT propagation was seen primarily on neurites, which became atrophied. This was accompanied by a concomitant loss of DARPP-32+ neurons, one of the main features of HD pathology. Finally, the location of mHTT aggregates was first identified in the cytoplasm and subsequently in the cell nucleus. It should be noted that the authors repeated the experiment using human pluripotent stem cells differentiated into neurons in which they confirmed the transsynaptic spread of mHTT from the R6/2 host tissue to human grafts, indicating that this was common to different cell types.

A final set of experiments was performed *in vivo* where WT mice were injected with HTTExon1Q72 and synaptophysin-GFP viral vectors into cerebral cortical layers. In this case, mHTT aggregates were detected predominantly in MSNs expressing GFP which were innervated by cortical projection neurons previously transduced with the viruses, suggesting an active role of cortical projections in mHTT propagation to striatal neurons. Post-mortem analyses of grafted hGFP-neurons in cortical areas of 4-week-old R6/2 mice further confirmed these observations.

The seminal work of Pecho-Vrieseling et al. (Pecho-Vrieseling et al., 2014) supported the hypothesis brought forward by Cicchetti et al. (Cicchetti et al., 2014) that mHTT could propagate transsynaptically between disease and healthy tissue. But exactly how mHTT is transported whithin neurons remains unanswered. To understand this, microfluidic culture devices have been employed in which neuronal somata could be isolated from their processes and other cell types. Using this system, it was shown that synthetic α-syn fibrils can be transported both anterogradely and retrogradely (Brahic et al., 2016; Freundt et al., 2012; Volpicelli-Daley et al., 2011), as well as to be released and taken up by second order neurons (Freundt et al., 2012). Similar observations have been made with Aβ42 (Brahic et al., 2016; Freundt et al., 2012), tau (Brahic et al., 2016; Wu et al., 2013) and HTTExon1 fibrils (Brahic et al., 2016). However, HTTExon1 fibrils showed limited anterograde transport, although retrograde transport efficiency was similar to that seen with α-syn fibrils (Brahic et al., 2016).

It has now been demonstrated *in vitro* that mHTT is able to disrupt vesicular and mitochondrial trafficking by recruiting and sequestering key elements of the axonal trafficking machinery, such as normal HTT, within aggregates (Trushina et al., 2006). This could explain the differences observed in the axonal transport between mHTT and other types of fibrils, and in particular the fact that, after retrograde transport, HTTExon1 fibrils accumulate intracellularly, while more than half of the α-syn and Aβ42 fibrils are released into the media (Brahic et al., 2016). It is clear that the properties of mHTT do not simply allow for it to be transferred between cells but that it is also capable of triggering aggregate formation using endogenous proteins within the recipient cell - and by so doing display prionic characteristics.

11.2 Tunneling nanotubes

Tunneling nanotubes (TNTs) are small entities that serve as a communication bridge between cells (Abounit and Zurzolo, 2012). Using adhesion proteins and fusion molecules (SNARE or viral fusion proteins), TNTs can change their configuration to merge to other cellular surfaces (Marzo et al., 2012). Neurons and various other cell types have the ability to produce these temporary and retractable protrusions which are made of F-actin strains and lipid bilayers containing organelles, plasma membrane components and ions such Ca^{2+} which are key to cell signaling (Smith et al., 2011). In normal physiological conditions, they have been noted to participate to cell development (Gurke et al., 2008), contribute to immune responses (Watkins and Salter, 2005), engage in regeneration processes (Wang et al., 2011) as well as facilitate electrical conduction between cells (Smith et al., 2011).

Pathogens and prion-like proteins can also hijack TNTs and for intercellular transport (Abounit and Zurzolo, 2012; Gousset et al., 2009) (**Figure 6**). This has been demonstrated in mouse catecholaminergic neuronal cells for α-syn (Saïda Abounit et al., 2016) and in both mouse catecholaminergic neuronal cells and mouse cerebellar granule neurons for mHTT (Costanzo et al., 2013). Furthermore, HTT and mHTT have been shown to form strong interactions with phospholipid bilayers, suggesting that they can drift on F-actin streams and lipid surfaces (Marzo et al., 2012). More specifically, α-syn fibrils taken up from the media are almost exclusively found embedded in endolysosomal vesicles (Saïda Abounit et al., 2016) within TNTs. In contrast, mHTT fibrils are identified in free forms within the cell cytoplasm (Ren et al., 2009) (**Table 2**) and their colocalization with vimentin hints to potential transport within aggresome-like structures (Costanzo et al., 2013). Although TNT formation can offer a defense mechanism for expelling material that the cell cannot digest/degrade – for example fibrillar amyloids – this system is not sufficient to completely restore the cell's health. Additionally, cells that contain pathological proteins produce more TNTs (Saida Abounit et al., 2016; Saïda Abounit et al., 2016; Costanzo et al., 2013), creating opportunities for pathological protein transfer and potentially facilitating the seeding process in naïve cells.

11.3 Exosomes and exophers

It has now been clearly shown that misfolded proteins can be found within extracellular vesicles and that they can be carried and delivered to a recipient cell using this means (**Figure 6**). The demonstration that this applies to mHTT as well has also been shown using exosomes extracted from fibroblasts derived from a severe juvenile HD case harboring 143 CAG repeats (HD143F) and which were exposed to differentiated neuronal stem cells derived from embryonic cortical mouse tissue. After 4 days of contact between the exosomes and the cultured cells, the internalization of mHTT was detectable. Similar results were achieved when HD143F-derived exosomes were incubated with SH-SY5Y cells, confirming the spreading capacity of mHTT via exosomes in various cell types (Jeon et al., 2016) (**Table 2**). Most strikingly, HD143F exosomes injected intraventricullarly into new-born WT animals led to the development of motor and cognitive HD-related behavioral phenotypes (Jeon et al., 2016). This study provided evidence that exosomes carrying mHTT could participate to disease onset/manifestation both *in vitro* and *in vivo*.

More recently, the *C. elegans* model has served to identify a novel vesicular entity capable of incorporating and extruding dysfunctional organelles as well as protein aggregates. This transporter was named an "exopher" (Melentijevic et al., 2017). Despite their larger size and the fact that they are born from a different genesis process, exophers resemble, in many ways, exosomes found in mammalian cells. They are released in a multiple-step process which includes protrusion, elongation and separation (**Figure 6**), emerging from the soma of different neurons, independently of cell division or cell death (Melentijevic et al., 2017). Their production is triggered by cellular stress, disruption of physiological conditions or, importantly, by the presence of IBs such as mHTT aggregates (Melentijevic et al., 2017). For example, the expression of aggregable HTTQ128 in the genome of the nematode causes impairments of the normal functions of chaperones, autophagy pathways, ubiquitin-proteasome systems and provokes the collapse of the integrity maintenance machinery in cellular elements. The accumulated stress increases the production of exophers in touch-responsive ALMR neurons expressing Q128 in this animal which in fact serves as a defense mechanisms to restore the cell's equilibrium (Melentijevic et al., 2017). However, the downside of exopher production is that they may, like exosomes, enable cell-to-cell delivery of insoluble pathogenic proteins (Melentijevic et al., 2017) (**Table 2**).

11.4 Endocytosis

Via endocytosis, the cells internalize several substances within the plasma membrane, which embeds them in lipidic vesicles and releases them into the cytoplasm (Mukherjee et al., 1997). The process begins with modifications of the plasma membrane, the generation of endocytic vesicles, which then matures into *early* and *late* endosomes, and finally leads to the degradation of the vesicle content through the fusion with lysosomes (Miaczynska and

Stenmark, 2008). There is now compelling evidence that proteins, such as α-syn, can be incorporated into cells via clathrin-dependent endocytosis (Oh et al., 2016) (**Figure 6**). Using undifferentiated and differentiated N2A cells exposed to HTTExon1Q44 and treated with various pharmacological compounds, clathrin-dependent endocytosis was identified to participate in mHTT uptake. In this particular study, HTTExon1Q44 fibrils were found in early endosomes of undifferentiated cells. This was observed as early as 6 hours post-exposure to the toxic material or in both early endosomes and lysosomes 24 hours post-exposure. At 48 hours, concentrations of fibrils were unchanged within the lysosomes, but were found at lower concentrations in the early endosomes (Ruiz-Arlandis et al., 2016) (**Table 2**). It was speculated that mHTT concentrations inside endosomes was lower because mHTT had been delivered to the lysosomes. In contrast, the stable concentrations of mHTT inside the lysosomes may have resulted from an equilibrium between the quantities of ingested versus degraded fibrils. It is also feasible, according to the authors, that this observation reflects the saturation of the lysosome degradation machinery. It has been noted that the fate of the same fibrils differed in differentiated N2A, where colocalization within early endosomes could not be firmly established (Ruiz-Arlandis et al., 2016). Rather, mHTT fibrils were present within lysosomes, perhaps testifying to the cell's attempt to eliminate toxic mHTT through lysosomal degradation (Ruiz-Arlandis et al., 2016).

The idea that the turnover of HTT and mHTT aggregates is dependent on the endosomal–lysosomal system finds supports in another study in which it has been reported that following transfection, free HTT accumulated in the cytoplasm and inside autophagosome-like vacuoles, while mHTT localized both to the cytoplasm and nucleus. The presence of mHTT in vacuoles modified the morphology of the cells, which appeared atrophied, further implying that endosomal-lysosomal-vacuolar pathway activation may be responsible for this type of cell death (Kegel et al., 2000). HTT and mHTT have also be shown to colocalize with late endosome and lysosome markers and this has led to speculation that this was due to the lysosome's capacity to mediate the secretion of proteins fusing with the plasma membrane through an active calcium dependent process (**Figure 6**). Endosome ablation, calcium chelator or silencing synaptotagmin 7 (lysosome-specific calcium sensor) inhibited mHTT secretion, providing evidence for the involvement of late endosomal/lysosome pathway in secreting mHTT and, in smaller amounts, WT HTT (Trajkovic et al., 2017).

11.5 Direct penetration of plasma membranes

Release and uptake are the basic elements of a prion-like propagation process. In order to dissect the mechanisms of transit between cells, artificially manufactured polyQ proteins were incorporated to the media of different mammalian cell cultures to verify and monitor their potential internalization, location after uptake and consequent toxic effects. Internalization of liposome-coated (4 hours post-infection) and uncoated fibrils (24-48 hours post-infection), characterized by 42 CAG repeats, were detected in both Cos-7 and PC-12 cells (**Table 2**). In this context, the presence of synthetic aggregates within the cytoplasm did not interfere with the physiological functions of the acceptor cells. To mimic the physiological expression of mHTT inclusions in the nucleus (Saudou et al., 1998) - which has been suggested to induce greater toxicity - the penetrance of the nuclear membrane was induced by the modification of the polyQ peptides by adding the molecular tag "nuclear localization signals" (NLS). Cell death was frequent in Cos-7 and PC-12 cells administered with F-LNS-Q42 or F-LNS-Q20 and was strictly associated with smaller sized fibrils (Yang et al., 2002), suggesting that the presence of polyQ into the nucleus is linked to high toxicity, independent of the polyQ length (**Table 2**).

A more elaborate study conducted in a wide variety of mammalian cells (Cos-7, HEK, N2A, CHO, HeLa) revealed that only one hour after contact, synthetic K2Q44K2 peptides were found within the cytoplasm, colocalizing with cytosolic quality control components in all cell types (Ren et al., 2009). Although their location was expected within the endosomal compartment (Lee et al., 2008), no colocalization with endosome, lysosome and autophagosome markers was revealed suggesting that fibrils are found free within the cytoplasm and are thus available to aggregate with other proteins including HTT (Ren et al., 2009). Transmission electron microscopy further uncovered that K2Q44K2 could reach the intracellular compartment by physically breaching plasma membranes (Ren et al., 2009) (**Figure 6; Table 2**).

The hypothesis of free Q44 fibrils interacting with HTT was more specifically investigated by assessing the aggregation state of cyan fluorescent protein (CFP)-tagged HTTExon 1 Q25 (CFP–HTTQ25) in HEK cells after infection with K2Q44K2 (Ren et al., 2009). CFP fluorescence in cells not yet exposed to polyQ fibrils showed a diffuse nucleocytoplasmic distribution, as expected of the soluble HTTQ25 fragment. Following incubation with K2Q44K2 fibrils, CFP florescence colocalized with the fibrils in distinct puncta, suggesting the recruitment of the Q25 soluble fraction into the aggregates. Using other forms of fibrils (non-fibrillar HTTQ18 and fibrillar HTTQ51) in the same cell culture conditions, cytosolic nucleation was induced by fibrillar polyQ peptides (Ren et al., 2009) (**Figure 6**; **Table 3**). This technique was used in several studies providing evidence for mHTT seeding capacities in different cell lines such as HeLa (Trevino et al., 2012) or human and murine neuroblastoma cells (Ruiz-Arlandis et al., 2016). Additionally, exposure of PC-12 - that can inducibly express truncated exon1 - with cerebrospinal fluid derived from postmortem samples of HD patients or living BACHD transgenic rats, showed that mHTT could trigger the aggregation process (Tan et al., 2015) (**Figure 6**; **Table 3**).

11.6 Additional mechanisms

The seeding process of synthetic mHTT fibrils has been studied in greater detail with bimolecular fluorescence complementation assays (BiFC) alongside time-lapse microscopy, allowing for the visualization of HTTExon1 oligomer formation using halves of Venus fluorescent proteins (Herrera et al., 2011). With this approach, the reconstruction of a functional fluorophore testifies to the dimerization of mHTT fragments. A strong fluorescence signal was detected in Q103HTT-Venus transfected human glioma cells (H4), while much lower signals were measured in H4 cells expressing Q25HTT-Venus. Dimers of 103QHTT-Venus constructs appeared 30-45 minutes after exposure, and some cells began to show larger aggregates after only 1 hour. Analyses at later time points, however, showed that all cells eventually died, indicating that both oligomers and IBs induced irreversible toxic effects. The cell-to-cell transmission potential of pathological mHTT exon1 fragment was further tested in H4 or HEK cells transfected with 103QHTT-V1 or 103QHTT-V2 plasmids and co-cultured. After three days, diffuse fluorescence revealed trafficking and, once again, the cell-to-cell transmission capacity of 103Q (Herrera et al., 2011) (**Table 2**). One important point to take into consideration is that the mHTT propagation does not always require cell-to-cell contact. For example, the media of HEK cells overexpressing GFP-mHTT-Q19 or GFP-mHTT-Q103 triggers spreading of non-pathological (Q19) and pathological length (Q103) polyQ in SH-SY5Y cells after 5 days of incubation (Jeon et al., 2016) (**Table 2**). This may indicate that, in *in vivo* contexts, mHTT could spread over extended distances and thereby exercising a toxic effect on remote cells.

Tau, α-syn and HTT Q50 fibrils can all be taken up by C17.2 cells and they are able to seed aggregation of intracellular tau RD-CFP/YFP, α-syn-CFP/YFP and HTT(Q25)-CFP/YFP respectively (**Table 3**). In particular, internalization of tau and α-syn fibrils has been shown to be mediated by heparan sulfate proteoglycans (HSPGs)-binding, which stimulates cell uptake via macropinocytosis. This internalization can be inhibited by heparin, chlorate and heparinase III (Holmes et al., 2013). It should be noted, however, that such uptake has not been reported for HTTQ50 fibrils, which suggests it may use a different pathway (Holmes et al., 2013). Similarities and differences in uptake mechanisms between proteins will have to be carefully taken into account when designing treatment approaches.

Mechanism	Protein form	Cell model	Observations	Reference
Transsynaptic propagation	Endogenous mHTT from R6/2 mice	*Ex vivo* mixed cortico-striatal cultures from R6/2 or WT mice	Propagation of mHTT from R6/2 cortical to WT striatal neurons Significant vulnerability of striatal neurons in comparison to cortical neurons	(Pecho-Vrieseling et al., 2014)
	Endogenous mHTT from R6/2 mice	Human ESCs and human iPSC differentiated into neurons transplanted into organotypic brain slices of R6/2 mice	Propagation of endogenous mHTT from murine host tissue to grafted hGFP neurons followed by progressive neurodegeneration of recipient hGFP neurons	
TNTs	Transfection with GFP-480-68Q (donor); mCherry (acceptor)	Co-culture of CAD transfected cells (68Q or mCherry) Co-culture of transfected	Transfer of GFP-480-68Q to both CAD and CGN neuronal cells via TNTs	(Costanzo et al., 2013)

| | | primary CGNs (68Q or mCherry) | | |

Vesicular transport

Mechanism	Treatment	Model	Finding	Reference
Exosome	HD143F-derived exosomes	Co-culture of HD143F and NSCs NSCs exposed to HD143F-derived exosomes	Spread of mHTT from HD143F to NSCs Spread of exosomes-containing mHTT in NSCs	(Jeon et al., 2016)
Exopher	Genetically-engineered expression of Q128	C. elegans	Q128 gene expression increases the production of exophers Exopher content, including organelles, protein and mHTT, is found in remote cells of the C. elegans	(Melentijevic et al., 2017)
Endocytosis	Fibrillar Alexa488-HTTExon1Q44 and/or polyQ44	Undifferentiated and differentiated mouse and human neuroblastoma cells (N2A and SH-SY5Y)	Internalization and intracellular localization of HTTExon1Q44 and PQ44 fibrils in both types of neuroblastoma cells Fibrillar HTTExon1Q44 uptake via clathrin-dependent endocytosis No mechanisms evaluated for PQ44 fibrils	(Ruiz-Arlandis et al., 2016)
Direct penetration of plasma membrane	Synthetic K2Q44K2 fibrils	HEK; HeLa; Cos-7; CHO; N2A	Breach plasma membranes by K2Q44K2 fibrils in all cell types tested	(Ren et al., 2009)
	Transfection with ChFP-HTTQ25 and synthetic K2Q44K2 fibrils	HEK	Recruitment of soluble HTT forms into IBs by synthetic K2Q44K2 fibrils in transfected HEK cells	
	Chemically synthesized Q42, NLS-Q42 and NLS-Q20 fibrils	Cos-7; PC-12	In the nuclei, smaller aggregates are more toxic than larger ones in both cell types tested	(Yang et al., 2002)
Unknown	Transfection with 25/103QHTT-V1 and 25/103QHTT-V2	Co-culture of H4 cells expressing 103QHTT-V1 and HEK cells expressing 103QHTT-V2	Polymerization and cell-to-cell transmission of HTT oligomers	(Herrera et al., 2011)
	Exposure to conditioned medium derived from GFP-mHTT-Q19 or	SH-SY5Y cells	Presence of exogenous mHTT protein (Q19 and Q103) within recipient SH-SY5Y cells	(Jeon et al., 2016)

GFP-mHTT-Q103 transfected HEK cells			

Table 2. *In vitro* **evidence of mHTT spreading capacities**. Abbreviations: CGNs, Cerebellar granule neurons; ESCs, Embryotic stem cells; GFP, Green fluorescent protein; HD, Huntington's disease; HD143F, Human fibroblast derived from Huntington's disease patient carrying 143 polyglutamine repeats; HEK, Human embryonic kidney cells; hGFP neurons, Human GFP positive neurons; HTT, Huntingtin; IBs, Inclusion bodies; iPSC, Induced pluripotent stem cells; mHTT, Mutant huntingtin; NSCs, Neural stem cells; NLS, Nuclear localization signals; PolyQ, Polyglutamine; TNTs, Tunneling nanotubes; V1, Venus protein half 1; V2, Venus protein half 2; WT, wild-type. Source (Masnata and Cicchetti, 2017).

Protein form	Cell model	Observations	Reference
Co-transfection with poly25Q EGFP and poly104Q c-Myc	Cos-1	Co-aggregation of normal-length and extended polyQ tracts into cell cytoplasm	(Kazantsev et al., 1999)
Co-transfection with poly25Q nucleolin EGFP and poly104Q c-Myc	Cos-1	Heterogeneous aggregates of 104Q c-Myc and 25Q-nucleolin- EGFP within cell nuclei Appearance of homogenous cytoplasmic inclusions with the expression of 104Q c-Myc only	(Kazantsev et al., 1999)
Transfection with 104Q nucleolin EGFP and 104Q c-Myc	Cos-1	Extended polyglutamine colocalization in both the cytoplasm and nucleus with the coexpression of 104Q nucleolin EGFP and 104Q c-Myc Interactions between polyglutamines causes relocation 104Q c-Myc into the nucleus	
Co-transfection of HA-HDQ20 and/or HA-HDQ32 with GFP-HDQ72	Cos-1	Elongated HTT polyQ fragments can recruit WT HTT	(Busch et al., 2003)
Transfection with CFP-Q25HTTExon1 and exposure to K2Q44K2 fibrils	HEK	Colocalization of CFP-Q25HTTExon1 with K2Q44K2 induces amyloid nucleation in a sequence-specific manner	(Ren et al., 2009)
Transfection with ChFP-HTTExon1Q25 and exposure to positive, neutral or negatively charged FITC-labeled Q44 fibrils	HEK	Induction of nucleation within the cytoplasm of ChFP- HTTExon1Q25 transfected cells by all three types of fibrils (i.e. positive, neutral, and negative net charges)	(Trevino et al., 2012)
Transfection with ChFP-HTTExon1Q25 and exposure to non-fibrillar K2Q44K2 aggregates	HEK	Reduced internalization of non-fibrillar K2Q44K2 and nucleation of cytoplasmic ChFP-HTTExon1Q25 in comparison to fibrillar forms	(Trevino et al., 2012)

Transfection with ChFP-HTTExon1Q25 and exposure to HTTExon1Q44 or Q44 fibrils	HeLa	Internalization of HTTExon1Q44 and Q44 fibrils into HeLa cells and nucleation within the cytoplasm ChFP-HTTExon1Q25 transfected cells HTTExon1Q44 fibril internalization is less efficient than for the Q44 fibrils	
Transfection with HTT(Q25)-CFP/YFP and exposure to HTT Q50 fibrils	Murine C17.2 neural precursor cells	Heparan sulfate proteoglycans-independent internalization of Q50 fibrils and nucleation with exogenous HTT(Q25)-CFP/YFP	(Holmes et al., 2013)
Transfection with ChFP-HTTExon1Q25 and exposure to HTTExon1Q44 fibrils	Undifferentiated and differentiated N2A	Seeding capacity of transfected HTTExon1Q44 fibrils with ChFP-HTTExon1Q25 in undifferentiated and differentiated N2A cells	(Ruiz-Arlandis et al., 2016)
PolyQ (KKQ30KK or KKQ40KK) oligomers	HTT14A2.6	Seeding of polyQ oligomers in HTT14A2.6 cells	
Exposure to media and lysates from induced HTT14A2.6 cells	Naïve	Media and lysates from induced HTT14A2.6 cells can seed aggregation in naïve cells	(Tan et al., 2015)
CSF from deceased HD patients	HTT14A2.6	CSF obtained from HD patients postmortem increase aggregate number in HTT14A2.6 cells	
CSF from BACHD rats	HTT14A2.6	CSF from living BACHD rats can seed aggregation	
Expression of PrDQ19, PrDQ54 and PrDQ92	GT17	Soluble Sup35 protein converts into insoluble aggregates following expression of PrDpolyQ pathogenic ($\geq$54 glutamines) proteins	(Goehler et al., 2010)
Transfection with Rnq1Q19, Rnq1Q54 and Rnq1Q91	GT17	Pathogenic polyQ tracts convert soluble Rnq1 into insoluble aggregates	
Transfection with HTT25Q-/103Q-GFP	74-D694	HTT103Q induce insoluble aggregates of Def1, Pub1, Rpn10, Bmh2, Sgt2, and Sup35 proteins HTTQ103 promotes it own aggregation and that of Sup35 and Def1 in different yeast strains	(Nizhnikov et al., 2014)
Transfection with HTT25Q-/103Q-GFP	BY4742 and 74-D694	Deletion of Def1, which normally enhances mHTT aggregation and toxicity, decreases selectively the amount of polymerized HTTQ103 and its cytotoxic effect in BY4742 cells	(Serpionov et al., 2017)

Table 3. *In vitro* evidence of mHTT seeding capacities. Abbreviations: BACHD, Bacterial artificial chromosome (BAC) transgenic rat model of HD; Bmh2, Protein BMH2; BY4742, Yeast strain; c-Myc, c-Myc tag peptide; CFP, Cyan fluorescent protein; ChFP, mCherry fluorescent protein; Cryo-ET, Cryo-electron tomography; Cryo-FLM, Cryogenic-fluorescent light microscopy; CSF, Cerebrospinal fluid; Def1, RNA polymerase II degradation factor 1; EGFP, Enhanced green fluorescent protein; FITC, Fluorescein isothiocyanate; GFP, Green fluorescent protein; GT17, Yeast strain; HA-tag, Human influenza hemaglutinin tag; HD, Huntington's disease; HEK, Human embryonic kidney cells; PolyQ, Polyglutamine; PrD, Prion domain; Pub1, Nuclear and cytoplasmic polyadenylated RNA-binding protein; Rnq1, Yeast prion protein;

Rpn10, Proteasome regulatory particle base subunit RPN10; Sgt2, Small glutamine-rich tetratricopeptide repeat-containing protein 2; Sup35, Yeast eukaryotic release factor 3; ; WT, wild-type; YFP, Yellow fluorescent protein. Source (Masnata and Cicchetti, 2017).

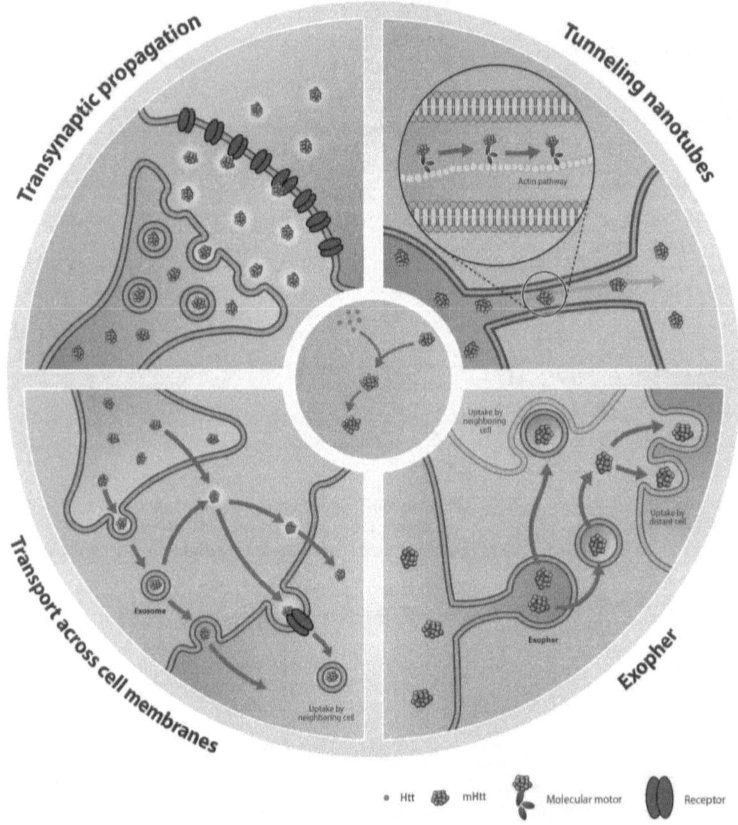

Figure 6. Putative mechanisms of mHTT spreading and seeding capacities.
Left upper panel: illustration of transsynaptic propagation of mHTT.
Right upper panel: transport mechanism of mHTT via tunneling nanotubes.
Left lower panel: mHTT can be released within exosomes or in a free form. After extrusion, exosomes carrying mHTT can fuse with the plasma membrane of a neighboring cell. Alternatively, mHTT can escape from the exosomal-vesicle into the extracellular compartment, with the same fate as the counterpart released directly as a free form. Finally, mHTT can be internalized by a recipient cell via receptor-mediated endocytosis or directly penetrate the plasma membrane.
Right lower panel: In neurons of C. elegans, mHTT has been shown to be contained within exophers, an entity which resembles mammalian exosomes. Released exophers may be incorporated by adjacent or distant cells or secrete their contents into the milieu.

12. Evidence for mHTT prion-like behavior *in vivo*

The injection of brain homogenates from patients affected with the prion disease CJD into healthy WT mice was one of the fundamental experiments performed to demonstrate the ability of the prion protein to propagate between different cerebral areas in a cell-autonomous fashion (Prusiner, 1982). The same experimental setup was adopted to test the prion-like capacity of pathological proteins contained in brain tissue from patients affected with AD or PD (Angot et al., 2012; Burwinkel et al., 2018; Clavaguera et al., 2013, 2009; Desplats et al., 2009; Faucher et al., 2016; Luk et al., 2012a, 2012b; Masuda-Suzukake et al., 2014, 2013; Meyer-Luehmann et al., 2006; Mougenot et al., 2012; Recasens et al., 2014; Ulusoy et al., 2013; Walker et al., 2002) (**Table 4**). Both AD and PD patients' brain homogenates injected into naïve rodents provoked (i) protein structural modifications, (ii) the recruitment, or seeding, of functional proteins into toxic aggregates and (iii) similar neurodegeneration to that observed in humans (**Table 4**). In subsequent work, different inoculum, including Tg mouse brain homogenates, purified oligomers, or synthetic fibrils, were also tested for prion-like capacity (**Table 4**). Synthetic fibrils, in particular, seemed to have a potent spreading and seeding efficiency since a single injection could cause significant detrimental effects (Luk et al., 2012a; Masuda-Suzukake et al., 2013; Sacino et al., 2014). For instance, either human or mouse recombinant α-syn fibrils when injected in the hindlimb muscle of premanifest TgM83 mice (PD mouse model that expresses the mutant human A53T α-syn under the mouse prion promoter) propagated through the brain to anatomically connected structures (Sacino et al., 2014). The intramuscular injection caused motor abnormalities and a decrease in lifespan. Furthermore, when the recombinant α-syn fibrils propagated within the brain, they formed pathological α-syn deposits (Sacino et al., 2014).

Giving the analogies among proteinopathies, similar techniques were used to assess the prion-like capacity of mHTT. For instance, the intracerebral injection of the lentiviral vector that carries HTTExon1Q72 into WT mice provided evidence that mHTT could propagate transsynaptically between cells in a healthy brain (Pecho-Vrieseling et al., 2014). However, this study did not investigate the outcomes of mHTT propagation with respect to neuropathological nor behavioral changes. To answer this specific question, fibroblasts from an HD patient (expressing 72, 143, and 180 CAG repeats), their derived exosomes and induced pluripotent stem cells (iPSCs) (expressing 143 CAG) were injected intraventricularly in WT neonatal mice (Jeon et al., 2016). Behavioral analyses were performed starting from 30 weeks of age for the animals injected with cells, and at 4 weeks of age for animals injected with exosomes. Sixteen weeks following injections, human mHTT positive aggregates were detected within striatal cells, providing evidence of human-to-mouse prion-like propagation of mHTT (Jeon et al., 2016). As early as 8 weeks post-transplantation, the mice started manifesting marked and progressive HD-like behavioral and histopathological phenotypes. More specifically, the animals displayed motor impairments, measured by the clasping test, and cognitive impairments, measured by the forced swimming test, all of which were associated with loss of DARPP-32+ neurons and gliosis (Jeon et al., 2016). These studies suggest that mHTT, as Aβ, α-syn and tau (**Table 4**), can behave in a prion-like fashion *in vivo*.

Inoculum	Injection site/administration site	Recipient/s	Outcomes	References
Alzheimer's disease				
AD patients' brain extract	Hippocampus, neocortex	APP-Tg mice	Seeding of Aβ resulting in senile plaques and vascular deposits (cerebral amyloid angiopathy) throughout different brain regions Presence of hyperphosphorylated tau AT8-positive axon in the proximity of the injection site	(Kane et al., 2000; Meyer-Luehmann et al., 2006; Walker et al., 2002)
	Tail veins	APP/PS1 mice	Spreading of Aβ seeds to the blood circulation and form vascular amyloid deposits (cerebral amyloid angiopathy) in the thalamic region	(Burwinkel et al., 2018)
Oligomeric Amyloid β-peptide (1–42)	Hippocampus (dorsal CA1)	C56BL/6 mice	Propagation in the surrounding region of the hippocampus Impairments in working memory tasks, but not spatial memory	(Faucher et al., 2016)
AD patients' brain extract	Tail veins	APP/PS1 mice	Spreading of Aβ seeds to the blood circulation and form	(Burwinkel et al., 2018)

			vascular amyloid deposits in the thalamic region	
Insoluble fraction of the P301S Tg tau mice	Hippocampus and cortex	ALZ17 Tg and C56BL/6 mice	Appearance of cerebral amyloid angiopathy Detection of pathological tau NFTs, NTs and oligodendroglial coiled bodies in ALZ17 Tg, and NTs and oligodendroglial coiled bodies in WT	(Clavaguera et al., 2009)
Human brain homogenates of AGD, PSP and CBD patients	Cortex	ALZ17 Tg and C56BL/6 mice	Spreading of exogenous tau to anatomically connected brain structures Observation of tau pathological accumulation typical of AGD, PSP, and CBD Widespread distribution of tau pathological species in a prion-like manner	(Clavaguera et al., 2013)
Blood of APPswe/PS1dE9	Joined blood circulation after parabiosis surgery	C56BL/6 mice	Detection of Aβ plaques, NFTs, signs of AD-like neurodegeneration and leaking vessels 12-month post-surgery	(Bu et al., 2018)

Parkinson's disease				
Symptomatic TgM83 mouse (mouse expressing the human A53T mutated α-syn) brain lysate	Cortex and striatum	Asymptomatic TgM83 mice, C56BL/6 mice	Development of motor abnormalities in asymptomatic TgM83 mice Deposition of LBs/LNs inclusions	(Luk et al., 2012b, 2012a; Mougenot et al., 2012)
AAV2/6 carrying human WT α-syn transgene	Substantia nigra	Sprague-Dawley female rats	Reduction of mouse life span Intracellular propagation of α-syn from a rat brain overexpressing human α-syn to naïve transplanted dopaminergic neurons in 3-6 weeks	(Angot et al., 2012)
Endogenous expression of α-syn	N/A	α-syn Tg mice	Propagation of α-syn to the healthy neuronal grafts	(Desplats et al., 2009)
α-syn amyloid fibrils	Cortex and striatum	Asymptomatic TgM83 mice	Widespread propagation from the injection site to several areas of the brain Recruitment of endogenous α-syn into LBs/LNs aggregates	(Luk et al., 2012a)
	Substantia nigra	C56BL/6 mice	Reduced mouse survival Recruitment of endogenous α-syn into LBs/LNs aggregates	(Masuda-Suzukake et al., 2013)

			Abnormal phosphorylated α-syn-positive structures at 15 months after inoculation	
	Substantia nigra, striatum, and entorhinal cortex	C56BL/6 mice	Propagation in the area far from injection site 1-month post-injection Detection of pathological hyperphosphorylated α-syn, hyperphosphorylated tau in presence of α-syn fibrils Impact of cognitive and motor behavior	(Masuda-Suzukake et al., 2014)
Insoluble fraction of DLB brain	Substantia nigra	C56BL/6 mice	Widespread detection of α-syn positive inclusions in regions distant from the injection site Detection of phosphorylated α-syn-positive structures	(Masuda-Suzukake et al., 2013)
Human purified LBs	Substantia nigra and striatum	WT mice, healthy non-human primate	Nigrostriatal neurodegeneration recruitment of endogenous α-syn	(Recasens et al., 2014)
rAAV expressing human α-syn	Left vagus nerve	WT Rats	Induced a strong expression of human α-syn in the medulla oblungata Propagation of α-syn pathology into other anatomically connected brain regions Pathological changes in neuronal morphology	(Ulusoy et al., 2013)
Human and mouse recombinant α-syn fibrils	Hindlimb muscle	Young TgM83	Motor phenotype in otherwise asymptomatic TgM83 2 months post-injection. Drastic reduction of survival Detection of α-syn pathology in the brain	(Sacino et al., 2014)

Table 4. Experimental evidence for the *in vivo* prion-like behavior of causative protein of neurodegenerative diseases. Abbreviations: α-syn, α-synuclein; Aβ, Amyloid beta; AD, Alzheimer's disease; AGD, Argyrophilic Grain disease; APP, Amyloid precursor protein; CBD, Corticobasal degeneration; DLB, Dementia with Lewy bodies; LBs, Lewy bodies; LNs, Lewy neurites; NFTs, Neurofibrillary tangles; NTs, Neuropil treads; PSP, Progressive supranuclear palsy; rAAV, Recombinant Adeno-Associated Virus; Tg, Transgenic; WT, wild-type. Table made by Maria Masnata.

13. Hypothesis and objectives

The laboratory of Dr. Cicchetti investigates many aspects of HD, in particular, her work focuses on understanding the contribution of the prion-like capacity of mHTT. Numerous reports now suggest that mHTT can propagate in a non-autonomous manner and recruit WT HTT into aggregates (**Table 2 and 3**). Furthermore, mHTT propagation is associated with behavioral as well as physiopathological alterations in various models (Babcock and Ganetzky, 2015; Jeon et al., 2016). For my PhD book, we hypothesized that mHTT possesses spreading and seeding capacity that may influence HD development. To test this hypothesis, my work aimed to investigate the prion-like characteristics of mHTT fibrils in *in vitro* and *in vivo* paradigms.

- *In vitro* paradigms were used to study the capacity of exogenous mHTT fibrils to be uptaken by 3 different human cell lines – SH-SY5Y, THP1 and iGABA cells – (spreading). Pathological changes, such as the increase in the number of apoptotic cells, morphological changes as well as the recruitment of endogenous HTT into insoluble aggregates (seeding) were analyzed.

- In the *in vivo* paradigm, we injected WT and HD mice with mHTT fibrils - in both CNS and periphery - to track propagation. A battery of behavioral tests and post-mortem analyses were conducted to identify phenotypic abnormalities as well as the effects on endogenous HTT.

Chapter 1: Demonstration of prion-like properties of mutant huntingtin fibrils

in both *in vitro* and *in vivo* paradigms

Demonstration of prion-like properties of mutant huntingtin fibrils in both *in vitro* and *in vivo* paradigms

Maria Masnata[*,1,2], Giacomo Sciacca[*,1,2], Alexander Maxan[*,1,2], Luc Bousset[*,4], Hélena Denis[1,2], Florian Lauruol[1,2], Linda David[1,2], Martine Saint-Pierre[1,2], Jeffrey H. Kordower[3], Ronald Melki[^,4], Melanie Alpaugh[^,1,2], Francesca Cicchetti[^,1,2]

[1]Centre de Recherche du CHU de Québec, Axe Neurosciences, 2705 Boulevard Laurier, Québec, QC, Canada; [2]Département de Psychiatrie & Neurosciences, Université Laval, Québec, QC, Canada; [3]Department of Neurological Sciences, Rush University Medical Centre, Chicago, Illinois, USA; [4]Laboratory of Neurodegenerative Diseases, Institut François Jacob, MIRCen, CEA, CNRS, Fontenay-aux-Roses, France

Equal contribution

^*Co-corresponding authors*

Correspondence to either:
Ronald Melki, Ph.D.
Institut François Jacob (MIRCen)
CEA and Laboratory of Neurodegenerative Diseases CNRS
18 Route du Panorama, Fontenay-Aux-Roses cedex, France, 92265
Tel: +33 146549378
Email: ronald.melki@cnrs.fr

Melanie Alpaugh, Ph.D.
Centre de Recherche du CHU de Québec
Axe Neuroscience, T2-50
2705 boulevard Laurier, Québec, QC
Canada, G1V 4G2
Tel: (418) 525-4444 ext. 42296
Fax: (418) 654-2753
Email: melanie-jeanne.alpaugh.1@ulaval.ca

Francesca Cicchetti, Ph.D.
Centre de Recherche du CHU de Québec
Axe Neuroscience, T2-50
2705 boulevard Laurier, Québec, QC
Canada, G1V 4G2
Tel: (418) 525-4444 ext. 48853
Fax: (418) 654-2753
Email: francesca.cicchetti@crchul.ulaval.ca

1.1 Résumé

Au cours des dernières années, plusieurs études ont suggéré que la protéine huntingtine mutée (mHTT) peut se propager dans les tissus sains tel un prion. Cette théorie reste cependant controversée. Pour aborder ce concept et mieux comprendre les conséquences de cette propagation sur la pathogénèse de la maladie de Huntington, nous avons étudié les effets de fragments N-terminaux fibrillaires humains de la mHTT (Q48) et de la huntingtine (HTT) (Q25) dans 3 modèles cellulaires et 3 modèles animaux distincts. Au cours des expériences *in vitro*, des cellules neuronales humaines (neurones GABA dérivés de cellules souches pluripotentes induites (iGABA) et SH-SY5Y) ainsi que des macrophages humains dérivés de THP-1 ont été incubés avec des fibrilles recombinantes de mHTT. Tous les types cellulaire ont incorporé les fibrilles recombinantes de mHTT et HTT, induisant des changements morphologique ainsi que la mort d'un certain nombre de cellules. Suite à l'incubation des cellules THP-1 et SH-SY5Y avec les fibrilles recombinantes, l'induction de l'agrégation a été observées. Au cours des expériences *in vivo*, les fibrilles ont été administrées à ses souris sauvages (WT) adultes via une injection corticale unilatérale tandis que les souriceaux R6/2 et WT ont subi des injections intraventriculaires bilatérales. Dans les deux cas, l'injection de fibrilles de mHTT (Q48) a entraîné des déficits cognitifs ainsi qu'une augmentation du comportement anxieux. L'analyse post-mortem du cerveau des souris WT adultes a révélé que la plupart des fibrilles avaient été dégradées/éliminées 14 mois après la chirurgie. Malgré l'absence de fibrilles, des changements des patrons d'immunomarquage de la HTT endogène ont été détecté. Un changement similaire a été observé chez les souris R6/2. Des expériences réalisées en parallèle ont toutefois révélé que des injections intraveineuses de fibrilles recombinantes entraînaient une réponse immunitaire. Dans leur ensemble, les données *in vitro* et *in vivo* indiquent que la mHTT administrée de façon exogène est capable de provoquer et d'exacerber la pathologie.

1.2 Abstract

In recent years, evidence has accumulated to suggest that mutant huntingtin protein (mHTT) can spread into normal healthy tissue in a prion-like fashion. This theory, however, remains controversial. To fully address this concept and to understand the possible consequences of spreading to Huntington's disease pathology, we investigated the effects of exogenous human fibrillar mHTT (Q48) and huntingtin (HTT) (Q25) N-terminal fragments in 3 cellular models and 3 distinct animal paradigms. For *in vitro* experiments, human neuronal cells (induced pluripotent stem cell derived GABA neurons (iGABA) and SH-SY5Y) as well as human THP-1-derived macrophages were incubated with recombinant mHTT fibrils. Recombinant mHTT and HTT fibrils were taken up by all cell types, inducing cell morphology changes and death. Variations in HTT aggregation were further observed following incubation with fibrils in both THP-1 and SH-SY5Y cells. For *in vivo* experiments, adult wild-type (WT) mice received a unilateral intracerebral cortical injection and R6/2 and WT pups were administered fibrils via bilateral intraventricular injections. In both protocols, the injection of mHTT (Q48) fibrils resulted in cognitive deficits and increased anxiety-like behavior. Post-mortem analysis of adult WT mice indicated that most fibrils had been degraded/cleared from the brain by 14 months post-surgery. Despite the absence of fibrils at these later time points, a change in the staining pattern of endogenous HTT was detected. A similar change was revealed in post-mortem analysis of the R6/2 mice. These effects were specific to central administration of fibrils, as mice receiving intravenous injections were not characterized by behavioral changes. In fact, peripheral administration resulted in an immune response mounting against the fibrils. Together, the *in vitro* and *in vivo* data indicate that exogenously administered mHTT is capable of both causing and exacerbating disease pathology.

1.3 Introduction

Huntington's disease (HD) is an autosomal dominant neurodegenerative disorder that progresses to death over 10 to 30 years (Tang and Feigin, 2012). During the pre-manifest phase, subtle changes in personality, cognition and motor control can be observed which, over time, lead to diagnosis based on motor features of the condition. Once manifest, HD patients exhibit progressive cognitive impairments that impact activities of daily living along with psychiatric disturbances that can evolve to frank psychosis and a worsening movement disorder. In the final stages, patients become demented and bedbound (Ha and Fung, 2012; Tang and Feigin, 2012; Walker, 2007; Zheng and Diamond, 2012). The classic neuropathological feature is a massive atrophy of the caudate and putamen which results from neuronal dysfunction and loss, especially of the MSNs. Progressive neuronal loss and atrophy is also observed in other areas of the brain including the deep layers of the cerebral cortex and it is likely that degeneration of cortical areas are responsible for the more critical cognitive and personality-related abnormalities seen in HD patients (Reiner et al., 2011; Vonsattel, 2008). Non-neuronal cell types are also impacted, with cell-autonomous changes in neuro-inflammatory cells such as microglia having also been described (Crotti et al., 2014). Importantly, HD is caused by a CAG repeat expansion beyond 35 in exon1 of the huntingtin gene which encodes for huntingtin (HTT), a cytoplasmic protein ubiquitously expressed and present both in humans and rodents, with a particularly high expression in the brain (Sassone et al., 2009). This leads to the production of a mutant protein (mHTT) with an expanded polyglutamine stretch (Bates, 2003; Zheng and Diamond, 2012).

Many proteins that play a central role in common neurological disorders, including α-synuclein, tau and amyloid have now been described to have prion-like properties (Brundin et al., 2010; Jucker and Walker, 2013; Soto, 2012). The concept of prions as disease causing agents was pioneered in 1982 with the seminal discovery by Stanley Prusiner that neurodegeneration in sheep and goats could result from exposure to a protein in an aggregated abnormal form, specifically to what has come to be known as a prion protein (Prusiner, 1982). It was demonstrated that this entity is capable of spreading and seeding pathology (Das and Zou, 2016). However, to be qualified as "prion", a protein must be capable of irreversible conversion of other normal proteins into a pathogenic form that can spread disease independently. From studying the proteins associated with neurodegenerative diseases, it has become clear that various factors influence how "infectious" a specific protein is. For example, the fibrillar form of α-synuclein is more toxic than the monomeric or oligomeric precursors (Pieri et al., 2012). Different cleavage products of proteins have differential abilities to be recruited and to subsequently seed pathology. Amyloid is the classic example of this with specific truncated forms such as Aβ 42 conveying far greater toxicity and infectivity than other similar structures such as Aβ 40 (Felsenstein et al., 1994).

From the initial reports, mHTT spreading/seeding was indeed highly debated, however, this theory is rapidly gaining support from both *in vitro* and *in vivo* experiments (Ast et al., 2018; de Calignon et al., 2012; Desplats et al., 2009; Hansen et al., 2011; Luk et al., 2012b, 2012a; Masnata and Cicchetti, 2017; Meyer-Luehmann et al., 2006, 2003; Ren et al., 2009). Despite the increased acceptance of mHTT spreading and seeding, the relevance of these phenomena in HD still raises significant scepticism; scepticism which is being further challenged by recent reports that mHTT with high seeding capacity is associated with greater neuronal toxicity in a Drosophila model of HD (Ast et al., 2018). To shed further light on these properties and their consequences, 3 distinct human cell models and 3 animal paradigms were used in which the impact of recombinant N-terminal HTT fibrillar fragments, termed HTTExon1 throughout the manuscript, were thoroughly investigated.

1.4 Materials and methods

1.4.1 Recombinant HTTExon1Q25 and Q48 fibrils

The expression and purification of human HTTExon1 with a 25 (normal) or 48 (pathological) glutamine stretch was performed, as previously described (Monsellier et al., 2015). Briefly, HTTExon1 was assembled in 20 mM Tris–HCl, pH 7.5, 150 mM KCl, 5 mM MgCl2, 1 mM ATP, 100 mM imidazole and 10% glycerol, at 37°C for 24 hours (hrs) (without shaking). HTTExon1 fibrils were centrifuged twice at 15,000 g for 10 minutes (min) and resuspended twice in phosphate buffered saline (PBS). The fibrils and BSA were labeled with ATTO-555 or ATTO-488 (ATTO-Tec GmbH Siegen, Germany, #AD 488-35 and # AD 550-35) N-hydroxysulfosuccinimide (NHS) fluorophore following the manufacturer's instructions using a protein to dye ratio of 1:2. The labeling reactions were stopped by the addition of 1 mM Tris pH 7.5. The unreacted fluorophore was removed by a final cycle of two centrifugations at 15,000 g for 10 min and resuspension of the pelleted fibrils in PBS. The amount of ATTO-555 or ATTO-488 incorporated was assessed by mass spectrometry. The samples were de-salted with 5% acetonitrile, 0.1% Trifluoroacetic acid (TFA) and eluted from a C18 reversed phase Zip-Tip (Millipore, Billerica, MA, USA, Cat# ZTC18M096) in 50% acetonitrile, 0.1% TFA. Peptide samples were mixed in a ratio of 1:5–1:20 (v/v) with sinapinic acid (10 mg/mL) in 50% acetonitrile and 0.1 % TFA and spotted (0.5 µL) on a stainless steel MALDI target (Opti-TOF; Applied BioSystems Foster City, CA 94404 USA, Cat# 4347686). MALDI-TOF-TOF MS spectra were acquired with a MALDI-TOF/TOF 5800 mass spectrometer (Applied Biosystems Foster City, CA 94404 USA) using linear mode acquisition.

Fluorescently-labeled HTTExon1 fibrils were fragmented for 15 min at 30°C in 2 mL Eppendorf tubes in a VialTweeter powered by an ultrasonic processor UIS250v (250 W, 24 kHz, Hielscher Ultrasonic, Teltow, Germany) set at 75% amplitude, 0.5 s pulses every 1 s. The nature of fibrillar HTTExon1 forms before and after fragmentation was assessed using a JEOL 1400 transmission electron microscope following adsorption onto carbon-coated 200-mesh grids and negative staining with 1% uranyl acetate. The fragmented fibrils were flash frozen in liquid nitrogen and stored at -80°C until use.

1.4.2 Cell lines and culture conditions

Experiments were performed in three different cell types: SH-SY5Y human neuroblastoma cell line, THP1 monocytes differentiated into macrophages, and iGABA high purity post-mitotic human neural cells derived from induced pluripotent stem cells (iPSC). The concentration of fibrils was selected based on a dose response curve of SH-SY5Y cells using MTT reduction as an indicator (**Figure 1.7c**). The dose used in our experiments (0.05 µg/µL e.g. 312 nM) was selected such that we observed sufficient toxicity without detrimental effects incompatible with long-term observations.

Incubation with fibrils

The SH-SY5Y (human neuroblastoma) cell line was cultured in Dulbecco's Modified Eagle's Media (DMEM) F12 (Sigma-Aldrich, ON, Canada, Cat #51445C-1000ML) supplemented with 10 % FBS (Sigma-Aldrich, Cat #F2442-500ML) and 1X antibiotic antimycotic solution (100 units penicillin, 0.1 mg streptomycin and 0.25 µg amphotericin B per mL) (Sigma-Aldrich, A5955-100mL). Cells were plated on gelatin (Sigma-Aldrich, Cat #G1393) coated 12 mm coverslips (Fisher Scientific, ON, Canada, Cat #12-545-81) in 24-well plates (Sarstedt, Numbrecht, Germany, Cat #83.3922.005). Twenty-four hrs post-plating, cells were exposed to 1 µL of 5 µg/µL mHTTExon1 fibrils (312 nM) or 1 µL of 1 µg/µL BSA (15 µM) (BSA, BioShop Canada, ON, CA, Cat #ALB999) for 3 days (Delorme et al., 2016; Gonzalez et al., 2014; Velez-Lago et al., 2013; Wojtecki et al., 2015) (**Figure 1.1a**).

The THP1 (human leukemic monocyte) cell line was cultured in DMEM (Sigma-Aldrich, ON, Canada, Cat# 56499C-50L) supplemented with 10% FBS (Sigma-Aldrich) and 1X antibiotic/antimycotic solution (100 units penicillin, 0.1 mg streptomycin and 0.25 µg amphotericin B per mL). Cells were plated onto uncoated 12 mm coverslips (Fisher Scientific) in 24-well plates (Sarstedt) and differentiated into macrophages by adding 100 ng/mL phorbol-12-myristate-13-acetate (PMA, Sigma-Aldrich, Cat# P8139-1MG) for a period of 72 hrs. Cells were then exposed to 1 µL of 5 µg/µL mHTTExon1 fibrils (312 nM) or 1 µL of 1 µg/µL BSA (15 µM) for 24 hrs (**Figure 1.1a**).

The iCell Neurons cell line (iGABA); Cellular Dynamic International, WI, USA)) were thawed following company guidelines (iCell Neurons User's Guide, Cellular Dynamic International). Briefly, cells were plated in complete maintenance medium (Cellular Dynamic International) on Poly-L-ornitine (Sigma-Aldrich, Cat# P4957-50ml)/laminin (Sigma-Aldrich, Cat# L9393-100UL) coated 18 mm coverslips (Menzel-Glaser, Dublin, Ireland, Cat# BB018018A1) in 12-well plates (Sarstedt, Numbrecht, Germany, Cat# 83.3921.005). The iGABA cells were treated 24 hrs post-plating with 1 µL of 5 µg/µL mHTTExon1 fibrils Q25 and Q48 for 3 days and untreated cells were used as control (**Figure 1.7i**).

Immunofluorescence for in vitro experiments

After treatment, SH-SY5Y cells were washed with 37°C DMEM F12 (Sigma-Aldrich) and 1x Dulbecco's phosphate buffered saline (DPBS) calcium magnesium (Thermo Fisher Scientific, ON, Canada, Cat# 14040133) and fixed for 20 min with 4% paraformaldehyde (PFA, Electron Microscopy Science, PA, USA, Cat# 19208) pH 7.3. Cells were washed (3 x 5 min) with 1X DPBS, permeabilized for 10 min with 0.5% Triton X-100 (Sigma-Aldrich, Cat# T8787-100ML) in 1X PBS, and blocked for 1 hr in 3% normal donkey serum (Sigma-Aldrich, Cat# D9663-10ML) in 1X PBS. Cells were then incubated with primary anti-Cleaved Caspase 3 antibody (Asp 175) (1:400, Cell Signaling, ON, CA, Cat# 9661S,) or anti-huntingtin (1:500, Millipore, CA, USA, MAB2168,) diluted in blocking solution overnight at 4°C, washed (3 x 5 min) in 1X DPBS, and incubated with Alexa 647 or Alexa 488 conjugated secondary antibody (1:500; Thermo Fisher Scientific, Cat# A32733 or A32723) diluted in blocking solution for 1 hr at room temperature (RT). Cells were then stained with Phalloidin Alexa 647 or Alexa 488 (5 µl per unit, Thermo Fisher Scientific, Cat# A22287 or A12379) for 15 min, washed (3 x 5 min) and finally incubated for 1 min with 4',6-diamidino-2-phenylindole (DAPI) nuclear stain (0.022%, Thermo Fisher Scientific, Cat# D1306). Both Phalloidin and DAPI were diluted in 1x DPBS. Coverslips were mounted on glass slides in Fluoromount G (Thermo Fisher Scientific, Cat# 00-4958-02). After treatment, THP1 cells were washed with PBS (3 X 5 min) and fixed for 15 min with 4% PFA pH 7.3. Cells were washed with PBS (3 x 5 min), permeabilized for 4 min with 0.1% Triton X-100 (Sigma-Aldrich) and 1 % BSA in PBS, washed with PBS (3 x 5 min) and blocked for 45 min in 1% BSA in PBS. Cells were then incubated with anti-Cleaved Caspase 3 (Asp 175) (1:400) or anti-huntingtin (1:500) primary antibodies diluted in blocking solution overnight at 4°C, washed with PBS (3 x 5 min), and incubated in Alexa 647 or Alexa 546 (1:500) conjugated secondary antibodies diluted in blocking solution for 1 hr at RT. Cell were then stained with DAPI and Phalloidin as described for SH-SY5Y cells.

Filter retardation assay

SH-SY5Y cells and THP1 cells were cultured as described above and plated in 6-well plates (Sarstedt, Cat# 83.3920.005). Twenty-four hrs post-plating, cells were incubated with 1 µL of 5 µg/µL mHTTExon1 fibrils (Monsellier et al., 2015) or 1 µL of 1 mg/mL BSA for 5 days for SH-SY5Y and 24 hrs for THP1 cells. Cell lysis was performed on ice, after one wash with PBS at RT, adding 150 µL of RIPA buffer (1% SDS) with 1% protease and phosphatase inhibitor cocktail 100x (Thermo Scientific, Cat# 78440). Samples were then sonicated for 2 X 10 seconds and resuspended with a 26G needle 5 times. After 30 min on ice, samples were centrifuged at 12,000 g for 5 min at 4°C. The filter trap assay was performed in triplicate with 50 µg of cell lysate diluted in PBS to complete a volume of 70 µL to which 30 µL of SDS:DTT mix was added (final concentration SDS: 2%, final concentration DTT: 100 mM). Samples were boiled at 100°C for 10 min, cooled to RT and the cellulose acetate membrane (Steriltech, WA, USA, Cat #1480025) was washed 2 X 5 min in 1% SDS in PBS prior to loading. After assembling the apparatus (HYBRI DOT Manifold, BRL Bethesda Research Laboratories, USA, Cat #1050MM), 100 µL of sample was loaded per well. After sample filtration, the membrane was washed 2X 5 min with 0.1% SDS in PBS in the filtration apparatus, removed from the apparatus, dried for 30 minutes, washed 3X5 min with 0.1% SDS in PBS and rinsed once in PBS to remove excess SDS. The membrane was then blocked with 5% BSA in PBS for 1 hr at RT, then incubated with anti-huntingtin (1:500, Millipore, MAB2166) or anti-huntingtin clone EM48 (1:500, Millipore, MAB5374) in 2.5% BSA in PBS-Tween overnight at 4°C. Incubation in secondary Azure spectra 800 goat anti-mouse antibody (Azure Biosystem, CA, USA, Cat# AC2135) was performed for 45 min and membranes were visualized using Odissey CLx imaging system (LI-COR, Bad Homburg, Germany).

In vitro quantification

All quantifications of photomicrographs were carried out with FIJI (ImageJ) on confocal images obtained using a 40X objective from multiple randomly selected regions across the entirety of the coverslip. Quantification of intracellular fibrils or conditioned media derived mHTT aggregates was performed manually and the position of fibrils/mHTT aggregates was confirmed using the orthogonal projection application of the software. The quantification of fibril size was performed using the "measure particles" function of ImageJ. The total number of cleaved caspase 3 positive cells was obtained using the "Cell counter" plug-in of ImageJ. The length of the longest projection emerging from the cell soma (defined as the primary neurite) was measured manually for each cell. The number of cells with secondary projections was counted manually. Filter retardation assay quantifications were carried out with ImageStudioLite software. The intensity of anti-huntingtin staining after exposure to HTTExon1Q48 is reported as percent change from the corresponding Q25 replicate (**Figure 1.4f**).

1.4.3 Animals

Three distinct animal experiments were conducted, two involving WT mice and one using the R6/2 model of HD. WT male C57BL/6NCrl mice were ordered from Charles River Laboratories at 6 weeks of age and were housed 3 per cage. WT mice received either intracerebral or intravenous injections. For the intracerebral protocol, mice were maintained for 14 months post-injection with behavioral testing occurring at 1, 2, 3, 6, 10, and 14 months. Behavioral tests performed were the open field, novel object recognition, light-dark box and the ledge test. For intravenously injected mice, behavioral measures were performed at 1, 2 and 3 months. Behavioral tests included the open field, Y-maze and light-dark box (all described below).

R6/2 ovary-transplanted WT females (B6CBA-Tg(HDexon1)62Gpb/3J) were purchased from The Jackson Laboratories. Pups were weaned as usual but underwent intraventricular injection of BSA, HTTExon1 Q25 fibrils or HTTExon1Q48 fibrils at post-natal day (p) 9. Genotyping was performed by polymerase chain reaction (PCR) analysis of DNA obtained from ear samples. Behavioral testing of treated pups began at 1 month and continued until 2 or 3 months of age. Each month, 1-2 mice per group were sacrificed to allow post-mortem analysis at multiple time points. Behavioral tests included the clasping test, cylinder test, grip test, open field, light-dark box, and Y-maze. Two animals per treatment group were sacrificed 1 hr post-injection and at the end of each behavioral testing.

All mice were maintained in a temperature and light-controlled environment (22 °C, a 12-h cycle) and all animal experiments were performed in accordance with the Canadian Guide for the Care and Use of Laboratory Animals, and all procedures were approved by the Institutional Animal Care Committee of Université Laval.

Intracerebral injections of fibrils

Eight-week old male C57BL/6NCrl mice (n=28/group) were deeply anesthetized by administration of 5% isoflurane, maintained at surgical plane with a dose of 1.5% isoflurane and kept warm with a heating pad. After the head was firmly fixed to a stereotaxic frame with ear bars, the skin was disinfected by swabbing 70% ethanol and chlorhexidine. A small portion of skin was cut with surgical scissors to expose the skull and permit the identification of bregma. Mice received unilateral injections of 2 µL Q25 or Q48 fibrils (1 µg/µL) into layer V of the motor cortex using the following stereotaxic coordinates: ML: -1.40, AP: ±1.60, DV: -0.75 ("Paxinos and Franklin's the Mouse Brain in Stereotaxic Coordinates, Compact - 5th Edition," n.d.). Injections were performed using a glass Hamilton syringe (Hamilton company, QC, CA, Cat# FSSP9718951) equipped with a 25 mm long 31GA needle and a bevel of 30° (Hamilton company, CAT# 7803-03). Following injection, the skin on top of the head was sutured with Vicryl sutures (Ethicon, PR, USA, CAT# J391H), isoflurane was interrupted, and the mice were placed in a recovery cage on a heating pad before being returned to their home cages.

Intraventricular injections of fibrils

Male and female WT and R6/2 pups (p9) were prepared as described above. Pups were then injected with 1 µl of solution containing 2 µg/µl of synthetic fibrils Q25 or Q48 or 1 µl of 1 µg/µL BSA bilaterally into the lateral ventricles using the stereotaxic coordinates ML: -0.90, AP: ±0.40, DV: -2,50, as previously published (Yang et al., 2016). Injections were performed using a glass Hamilton syringe (Hamilton company, QC, CA, Cat# FSSP9718951) equipped with a 25 mm long 31GA needle and a bevel of 30° (Hamilton company, CAT# 7803-03). Due to the young age of the pups, the skull surface was soft allowing the passage of the needle through the bone without requiring a microdrill. After the injection, the skin was fixed onto the skull with surgical glue (Vetbond, 3M, USA, Cat# 1469SB), the flux of isoflurane was interrupted, and the mice were placed in a recovery cage before being returned to their mother.

Intravenous injections in adult WT mice

Eight-week old male C57BL/6NCrl mice received intravenous injections of 3.5 µg of Q25 or Q48 fibrils (Q25, n=8; Q48, n=7) in 100 µL of isotonic saline every 2 weeks for 3 months.

1.4.4 Behavioral assessment

All behavioral tests were performed during the light-phase of the light/dark cycle and at the same time of the day throughout the study. The experimenter was blinded for the duration of the protocol. Prior to all behavioral testing, mice were habituated to the testing room for 12 hrs. The experimenter was present in the room throughout all behavioral tests, with the exception of the open field. All testing arenas were cleaned with 70% ethanol between animals. All behavioral tests were video-recorded and analysis performed off-line from the collected videos with the exception of the open field, which was automatically scored using PAS software and novel object recognition which was scored live.

Clasping

The clasping test is a standard measure of HD phenotype (Mangiarini et al., 1996). Clasping was analyzed by suspending mice by their tails 10/15 cm above the cage for 30 seconds. Two different parameters were assessed: 1) the time displaying whole clasping, defined as the retraction of all 4 limbs toward the abdomen and 2) a score of clasping intensity: 0 = no clasping, 1 = one hind limb retracted toward the abdomen, 2 = both hind limbs retracted toward the abdomen, 3 = all 4 limbs retracted toward the abdomen. We also measured the percentage of animals displaying whole clasping. This test was repeated every week starting from 4 weeks of age.

Open field

Mice were tested individually for 60 min in a PAS-home cage system consisting of a square Plexiglas arena (25" X 25") equipped with 16 X 16 photo beams that records beam breaks in real time (San Diego Instruments, USA). The distance travelled, average speed, number of rears as well as fine and ambulatory movements in the center of the field and the periphery were retrieved from the PAS software in 5 min bins. This data was used to calculate locomotor activity, anxiety related behavior as well as short and long-term memory (Bolivar, 2009).

Cylinder

Mice were placed in a raised transparent glass cylinder (diameter: 11.5 cm; height: 14 cm) for 3 min. Motor behavior was recorded by a camera placed on the bottom of the cylinder to observe how many times the animals touched the ground with the left, the right or both front paws. This was utilized as a test of gross motor function (Divito et al., 2015).

Ledge test

Mice were lifted and placed on the rim at one end of a clean cage. They were filmed throughout the time taken to walk from one end of the ledge to the other, and to descend down into the cage. Scoring was based on their footing: 0 – a mouse walked across the ledge with no troubles and lowered itself into the cage, 1 – a mouse lost its footing once or twice while walking across the ledge, 2 – a mouse was dragging its rear legs as it pulled itself across the ledge, 3 – the mouse fell off of the ledge or was unable to lower itself into the cage without falling head-first (Guyenet et al., 2010).

Grip test

We used an apparatus (Chatillon DFE II Series - Ametek sensor, tests & calibration) consisting of a grid connected to a force meter. Mice were placed such that all four limbs were on the grid allowing the mouse to grip the device. After placement, the experimenter gently pulled the mouse until the animal released its grip on the grid. The force meter automatically registered the force (measured in Kilogram-force (KgF)). This test was used to assess muscle strength (Castro and Kuang, 2017).

Light-dark box

The apparatus consists of two connected compartments of the same dimension (25 x 25x 25 cm), one black and covered to avoid light, the other open and transparent allowing the passage of light. Mice were placed one at a time in the dark compartment of the box. The time spent in the dark and the time spent in the light was measured as well as the number of head emergences from the door. The test has a total duration of 5 min and was recorded by a camera placed on the side of the apparatus. This test is used to assay the unconditioned anxiety related behavior as mice are nocturnal animals that prefer darker areas. However, when placed in a novel environment, they have the tendency to explore. The degree of anxiety influences the expression of these two competing drives permitting measurement of anxiety-related behavior (Kulesskaya and Voikar, 2014).

Y-maze

The Y maze apparatus is made of clear acrylic and composed of three equal arms measuring 32.5 cm in length, 8.5 cm in width and 15 cm in height. The walls of the maze are identical and opaque to prevent the utilization of visual spatial clues. Mice were placed one at a time in the middle of the maze and all four limbs entries were recorded by a camera for 7 min allowing the experimenter to be out of the mouse's field of view. A correct alternation was defined as successive entrance into each of the 3 arms, in any order, without re-entering one of the arms. Percent correct alternation was calculated as the number of alternation divided by the total number of entries minus two (Lalonde, 2002). The aim of this test is to evaluate short-term spatial working memory (Lalonde, 2002).

Novel Object Recognition

Mice were placed in an empty, transparent box measuring 40 cm x 25 cm after habituating to the behavior room for 1 hr prior to testing. Two identical glass rectangular prisms were placed at equal distances from the edges of the cage (12 cm). The mouse was placed between the 2 objects and allowed to explore the cage for 5 min. Two hrs later, the experiment was repeated but one of the rectangular prisms was replaced with a glass cylinder with floral decorations. The mouse was once again given 5 min to explore each of the objects. To measure the index of recognition, we examined the time spent observing: Object 2/(Object 1 + 2) (Zhang et al., 2012). To measure the index of demotivation: Object 1+Object 2 (2nd observation)/ Object 1+Object 2 (1st observation) (Antunes and Biala, 2012). Additionally, the total time the mouse spent observing the objects during both exposures was recorded. Time observation was measured as the amount of time the mouse spent with its head near the object.

1.4.5 Post-mortem analyses

Tissue processing

Mice were sacrificed at 1 hr, 4, 8 and 12 weeks post-intraventricular injection, 1, 2, 3 and 14 months post-cortical injection, or 3 months post-intravenous injection. All mice were subjected to intra-cardiac perfusion with PBS followed by perfusion with 4 % PFA under deep anesthesia with 1% ketamine (30 mg/kg) and xylazine hydrochloride (4 mg/kg). Brains were collected, post-fixed in 4% PFA overnight and subsequently stored in 20% sucrose in PBS for cryoprotection. For the intra-ventricular injection protocol, time points 8 and 12 weeks as well as all the other experiments, coronal 25 μm-thick brain sections were obtained using a sliding microtome (Leica Microsystems, ON, CA, Cat #SM 2000R), serially collected in anti-freeze solutions and stored at −20°C until use. For intra-ventricular injections, time points 1 hr and 4 weeks, coronal 12 μm-thick brain sections were collected using a cryostat (NX 70, Thermo Scientific) and mounted sections were stored at -20°C until use.

Preparation of plasma free of platelets

During sacrifice, ~1 mL of blood was collected by cardiac puncture into tubes containing 200 μL acid citrate dextrose and 350 μL of Tyrode pH 6.5. Tubes were centrifuged for 8 min at 600 g at RT. Platelet-rich plasma was collected and 1/5 of the volume of acid citrate dextrose and 1/50 of the volume of ethylenediamine tetraacetic acid 0.5 M was added to this, before the complete solution was centrifuged at 400 g for 2 X 2 min and at 1300 g for 5 min. The supernatant was then collected and centrifuged at 2500 g for 15 min to obtain the platelet-free plasma (PFP) for assessment of the antibody titre of animals administered fibrils by intravenous injections.

Immunofluorescence for in vivo experiments

Free-floating and mounted sections were washed in PBS (3×10 min), incubated in 3% H_2O_2 for 30 min, washed (3×10 min) and blocked with 10% donkey serum (Sigma-Aldrich), 0.01% Triton X-100 (Sigma-Aldrich) 0.5% BSA (Bioshop) and incubated overnight at 4°C with anti-HTTExon1 rabbit polyclonal antibody (1:1000, raised in Dr. Melki's lab using denatured HTTExon1Q45 as the antigen), anti-MAP2 (1:500, LifeSpan Bioscience, WA, USA, Cat# LS-B290-50, or 1:500, Sigma-Aldrich, M1406) and one of the following antibodies; anti-huntingtin clone EM48 (1:500, Millipore, MAB5374), anti-ubiquitin (1:100, Thermo Fisher Scientific, 13-1600) or anti-huntingtin (1:1000, Millipore, MAB2170). After primary antibody incubation, samples were washed (3 x 10 min), incubated with secondary antibodies (Alexa Fluor 488, 547, or 647 for the appropriate animal host; 1:500; Thermo Fisher Scientific or Jackson ImmunoResearch, ON, CA, Cat# 703-175-155) diluted in blocking solution for 2 hrs at RT, washed again, incubated with DAPI nuclear stain (Thermo Fisher Scientific) diluted in PBS to 0.022% at RT for 7 min, washed, mounted using Fluoromount G (Thermo Fisher Scientific) and stored at 4°C. For the immune-detection involving adult injected animals, mounted sections were kept in 70% Ethanol for 5 min, treated with Autofluorescence Eliminator Reagent (Millipore, Cat# 2160) for 5 min, washed 3 times in 70% Ethanol for 1 min each and then processed, as previously described (Neveklovska et al., 2012).

Enzyme-Linked Immunosorbent Assay

Antibodies against fibrils were tittered in PFP with an indirect homemade *Enzyme-Linked Immunosorbent Assay* (ELISA). Seven hundred and fifty ng of fibrils in carbonate 50 mM pH 9.6 solution were first coated in 96-well plates (Sigma-Aldrich, Cat# 3690) for 2 hrs. The plate was then washed 3 times with PBS 0.1 M with 0.05% Tween20 (PBST), blocked with 2% gelatin (Bio Rad, CA, USA, #1706537) in PBS 0.1 M for 2 hrs at 37°C and washed 3 times with PBST. One hundred µl of diluted PFP in 0.2% gelatin was incubated overnight at 4°C (dilution from 10^3 to 5.10^6). The plate was then washed 4 times with PBST and incubated with the secondary antibody conjugated with horseradish peroxidase: goat anti-mouse (1:25000, Jackson ImmunoResearch, Cat# 115-035-166) diluted in 0.2% gelatine for 2 hrs at RT. The plate was washed 4 times with PBST and then 3,3',5,5'-tetramethylbenzidine (G-Bioscience, Mo, USA, Cat# 00-4201-56) substrate was added for 15 min at RT. The addition of sulfuric acid 0.18 M stopped the reaction and measurement of the intensity at 450 nm was done using a multi-detection microplate reader (Synergy HT; BioTek, VT, USA).

Image acquisition and preparation

Fluorescent photomicrographs were obtained using a Zeiss Zen Imaging software linked to a Zeiss Imager Z.2 AXI0 confocal microscope (Zeiss, Oberkochen, Germany). All images were prepared using Adobe Photoshop CS5. When necessary, brightness and contrast adjustments were made. Panels were assembled using Adobe Illustrator CS5.

In vivo quantification

All quantifications were performed on pre-defined regions (prefrontal cortex, cerebral cortex, striatum, hypothalamus and hippocampus) across the entire brain. For the quantification of endogenous HTT by immunofluorescence, WT adult mice sacrificed 14 months post-surgery and R6/2 and WT littermates sacrificed at 12 weeks of age, were assessed. An entire series of sections encompassing the entire rostral caudal area of the brain was mounted on a slide and every third section of the slide was imaged with the distance between each section corresponding to a total distance of ~750 μm. In this quantification, we analyzed the area stained between different brain regions and treatment groups. Immunostaining was completed in two batches. To correct for differences between batches, data is shown as percent of Q25-treated WT mice. To further assess changes to endogenous huntingtin, the number of huntingtin aggregates were counted. These events were rare and we therefore analyzed the aforementioned regions of the brain through the binocular lens of the confocal microscope using the 20X objective, without sampling or acquiring pictures. Endogenous HTT is visible as a diffuse protein within all the cellular compartments. We considered any agglomeration of signal to be an aggregate. Finally, we detected EM48 and the HTTExon-1 in R6/2 mice injected with BSA, Q25 and Q48 fibrils by immunofluorescence at 12 weeks of age. For this quantification, the colocalization between HTTExon-1 and EM48 inclusions was quantified for Q25 and Q48-injected mice using the cell count plug-in in FIJI (ImageJ) photomicrographs. Colocalization was defined by overlap of different emission channels in multiple focal planes through each brain section.

1.4.6 Statistical analysis

For *in vitro* experiments, all statistics were performed using a students' unpaired t-test. For the *in vivo* experiments, two-way ANOVAs followed by Tukey's post-hoc tests were used for analyses of R6/2 and WT mice at a single time point, while one-way ANOVAs followed by Tukey's post-hoc tests were used when comparing three treatment groups of one genotype at single time point. Analysis of a single genotype across multiple time points was performed using a repeated measures two-way ANOVA, excluding animals that were not tested at all time points. A linear mixed-effects model was implemented to assess change overtime for two genotypes as a function of treatment group and genotype. Within-subjects variance was controlled for by including random effects of intercept and slope for each mouse. The model was estimated using maximum likelihood and contrast comparisons were performed to determine the effect of treatment and genotype at each time point. Analyses were performed using RStudio version 3.4.1 with nlme version 3.1-131. All data are expressed as mean +/- SEM. For all experiments, a significance cut-off of 0.05 was used. Graphs and statistical analysis were performed using the Prism software (v6.01; GraphPad Software, San Diego, CA) unless otherwise specified. For all t-tests and one-way ANOVA's, equal variance was confirmed by Fisher's test and where variances were unequal a Mann-Whitney test or Kruskal-Wallis test was used.

1.5 Results

1.5.1 Uptaken mHTTExon1 fibrils of human origin are toxic to multiple cells lines

To explore the spreading and toxicity of mHTTExon1, we opted to use recombinant HTT/mHTT fibrils which correspond to the product of exon 1 of the HTT gene. Fibrillar mHTT has previously been shown to be particularly toxic and prone to aggregate formation (Pieri et al., 2012). This makes this form an excellent candidate for understanding the potential of mHTT to spread and seed as it has the highest propensity to form aggregates. Prior to use, fibrils were imaged by electron microscopy. Both non-pathogenic Q25 (**Figure 1.7a**) and pathogenic Q48 fibrils (**Figure 1.7b**) were present in the solution and displayed the appropriate fibrillar structure (Monsellier et al., 2015). After confirming the presence of fibrils, a dose response curve was performed in a human neuroblastoma derived cell-line (SH-SY5Y) and 0.005 µg/µL was selected as the working concentration (**Figure 1.7c**). This concentration (0.005 µg/µL) fell in the center of the curve where minimal toxicity was observed. This intermediate concentration allowed us to limit effects on cell survival in long-term exposure experiments, while still maintaining a sufficient concentration to induce a cellular effect. SH-SY5Y cells were then incubated with HTTExon1Q25-ATTO488, HTTExon1Q48-ATTO488 fibrils, or BSA-ATTO488 for 72 hrs (**Figure 1.1a**). After exposure to fibrils, cells were fixed, immunostained for cleaved-caspase 3 as well as phalloidin to visualize the cell membrane. Using confocal microscopy, the presence of both Q25 and Q48 fibrils was identified within cells (**Figure 1.1b**). In agreement with previous findings by Ren *et al.* (Ren et al., 2009) quantification of the percentage of cells containing fluorescent puncta indicated that, while Q25 and Q48 fibrils were present within cells, there was a far greater number of cells containing Q48 fibrils when compared to Q25 fibrils (**Figure 1.1c**). Furthermore, cells exposed to Q48 fibrils had significantly more puncta per cell than did cells exposed to Q25 (**Figure 1.1d**). The size of the puncta within the cells did not, however, differ between the two conditions (**Figure 1.7e**). Fibrils had a toxic effect in both Q25 and Q48 conditions, but Q48 was significantly more toxic than Q25 fibrils (**Figure 1.1e**). This increased toxicity was unlikely to be secondary to the increased number of cells containing Q48 fibrils, as little to no cleaved caspase 3 activity was detected in SH-SY5Y cells containing Q25 fibrils. Contrary to this, 1% of Q48 fibril containing cells were undergoing apoptotic cell death (**Figure 1.7f**).

While neurons are among the most affected cells in HD, other populations, including microglia (Crotti et al., 2014), have been implicated in pathology. To determine if fibrillar mHTTExon1 also impacted different cellular populations, we exposed human THP-1 derived macrophages to Q25 and Q48 fibrils for 24 hrs (**Figure 1.1a and f**). Similarly to what was observed in SH-SY5Y cells, THP-1 derived macrophages incorporated fibrils from the media (**Figure 1.1f**). More cells contained Q48 than Q25 fluorescent puncta (**Figure 1.1g**) and more puncta per cell were present in cells exposed to Q48 than Q25 fibrils (**Figure 1.1i**). Macrophages did, however, differ from the neurons in few important aspects. The number of puncta per cell was higher in macrophages than in SH-SY5Y cells (**Figure 1.1d** and **Figure 1.1h**), the size of the puncta was larger in cells exposed to Q48 as compared to Q25 fibrils (**Figure 1.7g**), and there was no overall difference in the total number of apoptotic cells between Q25 and Q48 treated macrophages (**Figure 1.1i**). Importantly, there was still a difference in the toxicity of Q25 and Q48 fibrils, but this was only detectable in cells containing fibrils. In this population, there were also a higher percentage of Q48-containing cells undergoing apoptosis than Q25-containing cells (**Figure 1.7h**).

The similar findings we report in 2 distinct cell lines and previous publications (Ren et al., 2009), corroborates that Q25 and Q48 fibrils can be taken up and that they both can exert an effect on cells. However, there are a number of differences between cell lines and primary cultures. To confirm our findings in a more physiological relevant condition, iGABA human neurons derived from induced pluripotent stem cells were utilized. The iGABA cells were exposed to HTTExon1 fibrils or BSA for 3 days (**Figure 1.7d**). Similar to the cell line results, we observed uptake of fibrils from the cellular media (**Figure 1.7i**). Unlike the two cell lines, the number of iGABA neurons containing Q25 fibrils did not differ from the number of neurons containing Q48 fibrils (**Figure 1.7j**). Despite the similarity in the number of cells containing the two types of fibrils, there were still differences in cellular effects as cells exposed to Q48 fibrils were characterized by a significant decrease in the length of primary neurites (**Figure 1.7k**) and fewer cells depicted secondary neurites than cells exposed to Q25 fibrils (**Figure 1.7l**). These results confirm that fibrils can be uptaken from media into human cell lines in a number of different conditions.

1.5.2 Fibrils can recruit WT HTT into aggregates

To evaluate the prion-like capacity of human recombinant HTTExon1 fibrils, we assessed the state of endogenous HTT in SH-SY5Y cells. SH-SY5Y cells were treated with fibrils for 5 days (**Figure 1.2a**) and subsequently either fixed or homogenized. Fixed cells were immunostained for endogenous WT HTT to visualize changes in protein conformation (**Figure 1.2b**). To better facilitate quantification, the presence of aggregated HTT was assessed in cell lysates using a filter retardation assay. Increased aggregation of HTT was observed in cells exposed to Q48 compared to Q25 or BSA (**Figure 1.2c and 7d**).

To determine if this process was specific to neuronal-like cells, THP-1 differentiated macrophages were exposed to fibrils for 24 hrs prior to fixation and immunofluorescence detection of endogenous HTT (**Figure 1.2d**). This shorter treatment duration was selected for macrophages as they demonstrated faster uptake kinetics. After 24 hrs of treatment with Q48 fibrils, changes in the staining pattern of WT HTT were already clearly visible (**Figure 1.2e**). While colocolization and aggregation were apparent in the THP-1 cells, we selected to quantify aggregation using a filter retardation assay. Similar to the data obtained for SH-

SY5Y cells, we observed an increase in the intensity of WT huntingtin levels (**Figure 1.2f**) and aggregates (**Figure 1.2g**) after exposure to Q48 fibrils (**Figure 1.2f** and **7g**). Together, these two cell lines provide strong support for prion-like effects of Q48 fibrils *in vitro.*

1.5.3 Intracerebral injection of HTTExon1Q48 fibrils induces cognitive deficits and anxiety-like behavior in WT mice

To determine if prion-like properties of the abnormal HTT protein extended to *in vivo* conditions, WT mice received intracerebral injections of either HTTExon1Q25 or Q48 fibrils at 2 months of age (**Figure 1.3a**). Injected mice underwent a battery of behavioral tests at multiple time points (1, 2, 3, 6, 10, and 14 months) extending out to 14 months post-surgery (**Figure 1.3b**). The test battery included measures of motor function, cognition, and anxiety-like behavior as all of these behaviors are known to be altered in HD patients (Tabrizi et al., 2013). To assess motor performance, mice were tested in both the open field and ledge tests. No significant difference was detected between groups on either test at any time point (**Figure 1.3c and Figure 1.8a**). Mice were also tested for cognitive deficits using the open field and novel object recognition. In the open field, cognition was subdivided into short and long-term memory by assessing both habituation during one 60 min trial (intrasession) and between trials (intersession habituation) in the open field, respectively. No difference in short-term memory was observed 14 months post-surgery (**Figure 1.3d**). However, Q48 treated mice did demonstrate statistically significant impaired long-term memory at 10 (data not shown) and 14 months post-surgery (**Figure 1.3e**). Unlike the open field data, no difference in long-term memory was observed when measured using preference for the novel object (**Figure 1.3f**). Exploration time (**Figure 1.3g**) and motivation during the novel object testing phase (**Figure 1.3h**) did not differ between groups, which indicates that no motor confounds or differences in motivation influenced preference for the novel object. Finally, mice were also assessed for anxiety-like behavior using the open field and the light-dark box. In the open field, no change was detected in central ambulatory movements (**Figure 1.3i**), however, a mild increase in distance travelled in the periphery was observed after 10 months post-surgery (Interaction: $F_{6,118}=2.263$, $p<0.05$) (**Figure 1.3j**). The tendency to remain close to the walls is known as thigmotaxis and is indicative of anxiety-like behavior in mice (Kulesskaya and Voikar, 2014). The presence of an anxiety-like phenotype was further supported by an increased latency to leave the dark compartment at 6 months post-surgery (Time: $F_{6,120}$= 5.176, p<0.001, Treatment: $F_{1,120}$= 1.628, p>0.05) (**Figure 1.3k**). The anxiety phenotype was mild as it did not extend to a change in time spent in the light compartment (**Figure 1.3l**), exploration (**Figure 1.8b**), rearing (**Figure 1.8c**), or latency to first emergence of the nose (**Figure 1.8d**). The presence of cognitive impairment and anxiety-like behavior in Q48 injected mice supports the *in vitro* data showing toxicity and prion-like capacity of exogenously administered Q48 HTT fibrils.

1.5.4 Changes in the staining patterns of endogenous HTT in adult WT mice

In order to determine if the changes in behavior are due to human HTTExon1Q48 fibrils or their seeding propensity, post-mortem analyses were performed at different time points post-injection to track the localization of fibrils and to determine if changes in endogenous HTT were present. At early time points (1 month), fibrils were readily detectable using a fibril specific antibody (Monsellier et al., 2015) (**Figure 1.4a**). At later time points (3 months), fibrils became progressively more difficult to identify (**Figure 1.4b**) and were no longer detectable for HTTExon1Q25 by 14 months post-surgery (**Figure 1.4c**). To ensure that the staining observed was specific to the fibrils and to exclude the possibility of cross-reactivity with endogenous HTT, non-injected WT mice were also immunostained with the anti-exon 1 antibody and no punctate staining was present (**Figure 1.4d**). Given that the fibrils are mostly absent from the brain at the time points where behavioral changes were detected, it was particularly important to understand if HTTExon1Q48 fibrils were capable of inducing changes in the staining pattern of endogenous HTT. Interestingly, a change in the amount of positive HTT signal was detected between groups, with HTTExon1Q48 injected mice having reduced signal compared to their Q25 injected counterparts 14 months post-surgery (**Figure 1.4e**). These changes reached statistical significance in the prefrontal cortex (**Figure 1.4f**), although the more posterior cortical regions also showed a trend towards a decrease (data not shown). The changes in behavior and endogenous HTT staining patterns, even after the clearance of the fibrils, are consistent with mHTTExon1 fibrils possessing prion-like behavior.

1.5.5 Injection of HTTExon1Q48 fibrils precipitates disease in the R6/2 mouse model of
HD

Although experiments conducted in adult WT mice show that exogenous HTTExon1 fibrils
have seeding propensity, the behavioral impairments observed were subtle and took several
months to manifest. In a second set of experiments, mHTT fibrils or BSA, as a non-toxic
protein control, were injected bilaterally into the lateral ventricle of R6/2 and WT pups 9
days after birth (**Figure 1.5a**). The R6/2 model of HD has a very rapid disease course
(Mangiarini et al., 1996), therefore mice were followed for much less time (12 weeks)
(**Figure 1.5b**) than the aforementioned adult WT animals (14 months). HD mice underwent
a battery of motor and non-motor tests, similar to what was performed for WT animals.
Differences in performance between R6/2 mice injected HTTExon1Q25, HTTExon1Q48 or
BSA were detected as early as 4 weeks of age on the clasping test (**Figure 1.5c-d**). At this
age, mice injected with HTTExon1Q48 fibrils had an increased average clasping score which
was maintained until 12 weeks of age. At later time points, this difference was less striking
as the prevalence of clasping behavior increased in Q25 and BSA-injected controls as the
disease progressed (**Figure 1.5c**). While the difference between groups diminished over time
for clasping scores, the difference between groups for time spent clasping increased (**Figure
1.5e**), with HTTExon1Q48-injected mice displaying a highly statistically significant
difference at 12 weeks of age (**Figure 1.5f**). Increased motor impairment was not present in
the cylinder test (**Figure 1.9a**) or grip test (**Figure 1.9b**) although HTTExon1Q48-injected
mice did display a slight increase in the number of wall contacts at 8 weeks of age (**Figure
1.9a**). This phenotype was transitory and no difference between any groups was observed at
4 or 12 weeks of age. A subtle motor phenotype was, however, observed in the open field at
4 weeks of age. Male R6/2 mice that were injected with HTTExon1Q48 moved less in the
last 5 min of testing, which is likely due to increased motor fatigue in the later time points in
this 60 min test (Interaction: $F_{2,42}=5.10$, $p<0.05$) (**Figure 1.5g**). No such difference was
observed in female mice (**Figure 1.5h**). In contrast to the results in adult WT mice, no
changes in intersession or intrasession habituation were observed between R6/2 mice injected
with HTTExon1Q48 fibrils and with HTTExon1Q25 fibrils (**Figure 1.5g and h**). However,
there was a difference in cognitive performance between WT littermates injected with
HTTExon1Q48 and 25 fibrils in short-term memory at the 4-week time point (Interaction:

$F_{2,85}$=4.117, p<0.05) (**Figure 1.5i**) and long-term memory at the 8-week time point (Genotype: $F_{1,74}$=12.83, p<0.001, Treatment: $F_{2,74}$=3.152 p<0.05) (**Figure 1.5j**). In both the WT and R6/2 groups, BSA treated mice demonstrated a transient cognitive impairment at 4 weeks (**Figure 1.5i**) which was lost by 8 weeks of age (**Figure 1.5j**). This transient impairment may be the result of an exaggerated immune response to the presence of BSA in the brain, as previously reported (Habicht and Terres, 1966). We additionally observed a lower activity change ratio in Q48-injected R6/2 mice at the 8-week time point. Generally, this is indicative of improved memory but the extreme motor phenotype of R6/2 mice suggests that this decrease could instead be caused by motor fatigue in these animals. In a second well-validated cognitive test, the Y-maze, no change in working memory was observed at the 4-week time point where the decrease in distance travelled was evident. At later time points, R6/2 mice injected with HTTExon1Q48 had a reduced percentage of correct entries as compared to BSA-injected R6/2 mice and Q48-injected WT littermates (Genotype: $F_{1,55}$=13.54, p<0.001, Treatment: $F_{2,55}$ = 3.553 p<0.05) (**Figure 1.9c**). Q25-injected R6/2 mice did not significantly differ from either BSA or Q48-injected R6/2 mice. These mice appeared to be half-way between the two treatment groups, suggesting that Q25 may slightly impair cognition at this time point, but that Q48 has a more severe effect. This was the only test where Q25 appeared to exacerbate disease in R6/2 mice.

Anxiety-like behavior demonstrated premature manifestation in R6/2 mice injected with HTTExon1Q48 fibrils with these mice displaying increased anxiety-like behavior as compared to HTTExon1Q25 and BSA-injected mice which displayed decreased anxiety-like behavior at 8 and 12 weeks (**Figure 1.5k**). The performance of Q25 and BSA-injected mice is consistent with the progression of anxiety-like behavior reported in previous studies (Bissonnette et al., 2013). At 8 weeks of age, the difference between time spent in the light box by HTTExon1Q25 and HTTExon1Q48 was significant as assessed by Two-way ANOVA (**Figure 1.5l**). If all time points were considered in the analysis, both BSA and Q25 significantly differed from Q48-injected R6/2 mice. Anxiety-like performance was additionally measured using a second parameter, namely the time at which the head of the mouse enters the light box. This measure was consistent with the time spent in the light box with HTTExon1Q25, relative to HTTExon1Q48, showing a significant reduction latency to emerge at all time points (**Figure 1.5m**). This difference was preserved up to 12-weeks of age (end of the experiment) where BSA and HTTExon1Q25-injected mice both displayed a decreased latency as compared to Q48 injected mice (**Figure 1.5n**).

1.5.6 Exogenous HTTExon1Q48 fibrils colocalize with endogenous mHTT in R6/2 mice

The rapid disease course of R6/2 mice obliged us to conduct the post-mortem analysis 3 months post-surgery. However, this earlier time point increased the detectability of fibrils within animal brains, as the majority of fibrils were not cleared from the central nervous system prior to this time point. Furthermore, the presence of N-terminal mHTT likely increases the seeding propensity of exogenous HTTExon1 fibrils. This was assessed by immunodetection of endogenous mHTT with the EM48 antibody and fibrils with the anti-HTTExon1 antibody. Double immunofluorescence measurements demonstrated lack of colocalization of exogenous HTTExon1 fibrils and endogenous HTT in WT (**Figure 1.10a**). In contrast, colocalization was evident in R6/2 mice treated with HTTExon1Q25 or Q48 fibrils by 4 weeks of age (**Figure 1.10b**). Colocalization cannot be an artifact resulting from poor antibody specificity as it is only observed in R6/2 mice that were treated with fibrils. We nonetheless performed a number of antibody controls. First, to confirm that EM48 does not detect WT HTT, non-injected WT mice were immunostained with EM48 and no signal was detected. Similarly, the specificity of the antibody used to detect fibrils was confirmed by immunostaining in non-injected R6/2 mice. This control further demonstrated the absence of positive signal (**Figure 1.11a**). Absence of colocalization in Q25 and Q48 injected WT mice suggests that there was no cross-reactivity between fibrils and endogenous mHTT. We further used ubiquitin as a second antibody to detect endogenous mHTT aggregates in R6/2 mice, as previously described (Bayram-Weston et al., 2016). The same non-injected controls performed for EM48 were also done for ubiquitin (**Figure 1.11b**) and, they again, confirmed antibody specificity. After confirming specificity, WT and R6/2 mice were incubated with anti-ubiquitin. The absence of colocalization between ubiquitin staining and fibrils in Q48-treated WT mice and the presence of colocalization in Q48-treated R6/2 mice further validated the results obtained with EM48 (**Figure 1.11c**).

At the endpoint of this experiment, fibrillar puncta were readily detected in all fibril-treated groups (**Figure 1.6a**). R6/2 mice had more fibrils remaining in the brain 12 weeks after injection as compared to WT mice (**Figure 1.6b and c**). The cortex and hippocampus displayed the most striking differences, although an overall effect of genotype was detected in mice (WT and R6/2) exposed to HTTExon1Q25 fibrils (Genotype: $F_{1,40}=39.93$, $p<0.0001$) (**Figure 1.6b**). Whereas the cortex, striatum and hypothalamus exhibited the greatest difference (Interaction: $F_{4,40}=5.185$, $p<0.01$) in WT and R6/2 mice injected with HTTExon1Q48 fibrils (**Figure 1.6c**), the localization of mHTT puncta also differed. In WT mice, most fibrils were detected outside of cells, while in R6/2 mice fibrils were most often identified within MAP2$^+$ cells. This was not the case for HTTExon1Q25 fibrillar puncta, which were equally found inside and outside the MAP2$^+$ cells in WT and R6/2 mice (**Figure 1.12a**). Astrocytes and microglia were also assessed for the presence of fibrils but none were detected in either cell type, genotype or treatment condition. When Q25 fibrils were compared to Q48 fibrils within one genotype, puncta were less frequently seen in WT mice that were injected with HTTExon1Q25 than those that received the Q48 fibrillar counterpart (**Figure 1.6d**), suggesting that exogenous HTTExon1Q25 are processed (e.g. cleared or degraded) to a much higher extent than HTTExon1Q48 fibrils in the cortex (Interaction: $F_{4,40}=5.106$, $p<0.01$) (**Figure 1.6e**). A similar pattern of clearance was observed in R6/2 mice (**Figure 1.6f**). Interestingly, the number of exogenous HTTExon1Q48 puncta was significantly higher than that of HTTExon1Q25 puncta in the striatum of R6/2 animals (Fibrils: $F_{1,40}=8.359$, $p<0.01$; Region: $F_{4,40}=7.877$, $p<0.0001$) (**Figure 1.6g**). The seeding capacity of exogenous HTTExon1 was subsequently evaluated by quantifying exogenous and endogenous mHTT aggregates colocalization in R6/2 mice. Regions with the highest number of exogenous puncta tend to display more aggregations (Interaction: $F_{4,39}=2.727$, $p<0.05$) (**Figure 1.6h**). This was particularly evident in the striatum where a significantly higher colocalization was observed in mice injected with HTTExon1Q48 compared to HTTExon1Q25 fibrils (**Figure 1.6i**).

While increased colocalization between exogenous fibrillar and endogenous mHTT indicates that two pathological proteins may interact, true seeding requires interaction between a WT soluble protein and mutant seeds. Consequently, we assessed if the presence of fibrillar HTTExon1Q25 and Q48 could alter the staining pattern of endogenous HTT. To do this, we evaluated signal intensity and aggregation in multiple brain regions and found that both measures were impacted by administration of Q48 fibrils. HTT signal intensity was significantly decreased in Q48 treated mice in the hippocampus, cortex and striatum (Treatment hippocampus: $F_{2,22}$=7.283, p<0.0037; Treatment cortex: $F_{2,24}$=7.633, p<0.01; Treatment striatum: $F_{2,25}$=9.435, p<0.001) (**Figure 1.12c, d and e**). In the hippocampus, WT mice injected with HTTExon1Q48 depicted a strong trend towards a decrease compared to HTTExon1Q25 treated mice (p=0.0529) (**Figure 1.12b and c**), while R6/2 mice injected with HTTExon1Q48 displayed a significant reduction in signal intensity compared to BSA treated mice and a strong trend towards a decrease compared to Q25 treated mice (p=0.0586) in the hippocampus (**Figure 1.12c**). In the cortex, no treatment differences were observed in WT mice but Q48 treated R6/2 mice had significantly reduced signal compared to both Q25 and BSA treated mice (**Figure 1.12d**). HTTExon1Q48 treated WT and R6/2 mice displayed significantly decreased endogenous HTT signal intensity as compared to BSA mice (**Figure 1.12e**). In this region, the Q25 had intermediary signal levels, which did not differ from either BSA or Q48 treated animals. WT HTT aggregates were quantified in WT and R6/2 mice treated with Q25 and Q48 fibrils, however aggregates were only detected in WT and R6/2 mice treated with Q48 (**Figure 1.12f**). These aggregates were observed throughout the brains (**Figure 1.12g**). Together, these changes in WT huntingtin staining provide strong evidence for an alteration of the WT protein distribution by Q48 fibrils.

1.5.7 Peripheral injection of mHTTExon1 fibrils initiates an immune response

Both intracerebral and intraventricular infusion of exogenous mHTT fibrils is sufficient to induce a behavioral phenotype and a redistribution of endogenous HTT. To determine whether the behavioral phenotypes we observed upon injection of exogenous fibrillar HTTExon1 are due to their administration within the central nervous system, WT mice were injected intravenously HTTExon1Q25 and Q48 fibrils every 2 weeks for 3 months (**Figure 1.13a**). Mice underwent a battery of behavioral tests each month to assess motor performance, cognition and anxiety-like behavior. Motor performance was assessed using distance travelled in the open field (**Figure 1.13b**), cognition was assessed by intersession habituation in the open field (**Figure 1.13c**) and spontaneous alternation in the Y-maze (**Figure 1.13d**). Anxiety-like behavior was measured using the light-dark box (**Figure**

1.13e). No behavioral changes were observed through any test at any time point. The absence of phenotypic changes may be explained by an increased immune response that was observed in mice injected with HTTExon1Q48 fibrils (**Figure 1.13f**).

1.6 Discussion

We utilized multiple cellular and animal models to demonstrate that exogenous fibrillar mHTTExon1 is taken up, transported and seeds pathology within the brain in a manner similar to prions. We established that multiple cell types take up toxic HTTExon1 fibrils. Uptake is accompanied by the aggregation of endogenous HTT in SH-SY5Y cells, THP-1 derived macrophages and iGABA human neurons derived from induced pluripotent stem cells. While all 3 cell models displayed many common features, there were also some notable differences. Firstly, each cell line incorporated fibrils to different extents over different time scales. iGABA cells took up exogenous fibrillar HTTExon1Q25 or Q48 to the least extent (with only approximately 0.3% of cells containing puncta after 3 days of exposure). This figure was 5% and 20% for SH-SY5Y and THP-1 derived macrophages exposed to HTTExon1Q25 or Q48, respectively. The similarity between THP-1 and SH-SY5Y cells, as compared to iGABA, suggests that higher uptake may be a feature of mitotic cell lines, in agreement with previous reports (Ruiz-Arlandis et al., 2016), although we did observe the phenomenon in THP1 cells which are also post-mitotic. The reason why cells exposed to HTTExon1Q25 or Q48 do not contain the same number of puncta may be due to a better processing of HTTExon1Q25 compared to HTTExon1Q48. Indeed, we previously showed, using FTIR spectroscopy, that the two fibrillar assemblies exhibit structural differences (Monsellier et al., 2015).

Although HTTExon1Q25 and Q48 fibrils were taken up by iGABA cells to a similar extent, higher stress levels were observed upon fibrillar HTTExon1Q48 uptake. Interestingly, the two neuron-like cells exhibited 1 or 2 puncta upon exposure to fibrillar HTTExon1 while macrophages had 30+ much smaller puncta than those in neuronal cells. It is perhaps not overly surprising that a macrophage cell line attempts to degrade exogenous proteins to a greater degree than do neuronal cell lines. What is more striking, however, is that despite the differences in the processing of the fibrils, both neuronal and macrophage cell lines displayed increased aggregation of endogenous HTT, although at a much faster rate in macrophages. It is possible that the faster uptake kinetics and increased ability to degrade fibrils that characterizes macrophages also favors the interaction of endogenous and exogenous HTT and better seeding. Regardless, the filter retardation assay (refer to **Figure 1.2**) provides the first evidence that exogenous HTTExon1 fibrils seed the aggregation of endogenous HTT. Previous reports demonstrated seeding in transfected cells expressing high levels of endogenous HTT (Monsellier et al., 2015; Ren et al., 2009; Ruiz-Arlandis et al., 2016).

To determine whether what we observed *in vitro* applies to more complex systems, adult WT mice received exogenous fibrillar HTTExon1 intracortical injections. A single 2 µg dose of exogenous fibrils was sufficient to trigger a behavioral phenotype. However, the induction of a phenotype required a longer period of time than was previously shown after injection of iPSCs expressing mHTT (Jeon et al., 2016). Aside from the nature of HTT, there were other important factors that differed in the two protocols such as the age of the animals and site of administration (Akhtar et al., 2011).

A particularly salient finding in the WT adult background is the presence of behavioral and biochemical changes that persist beyond the presence of fibrils. Indeed, by 16 months of age, mice still displayed increased anxiety-like behavior, impaired cognition, and changes in the staining pattern of endogenous HTT even though the fibrils were no longer detectable. This indicates a sustainable and irreversible change triggered HTTExon1 fibrils. The decreased endogenous HTT immunodetection suggests that the persistent change caused by HTTExon1 fibrils may involve endogenous HTT. Interestingly, the changes in endogenous HTT state were most apparent in the vicinity of the cortical injection even though the striatum is the most affected region in HD. Although the regions with significant changes in endogenous HTT levels did not match with the pattern or regional susceptibility typical of HD pathology, the behavioral changes are consistent with typical disease manifestation. While the motor symptoms are the hallmark of HD and are necessary for the diagnosis of disease onset, they are not generally the first symptoms that present. In most patients and animal models of HD, cognitive deficits and anxiety-like behavior precede the onset of motor symptoms (Epping et al., 2016; Williams et al., 2015). It is therefore probable that at later stages, a motor phenotype may have begun to emerge. It is also possible that the motor phenotype was less evident at late time points due to the advanced age of the mice and the decrease in motor acuity that accrues as part of the aging process (Allen et al., 2011).

Studies in R6/2 mice further demonstrated the capacity of fibrillar HTTExon1Q48 to precipitate disease phenotype. In this second set of experiments, we included BSA as a negative control to determine if the injection of Q25 had any behavioral consequences. This control revealed that there were no significant differences between BSA-injected and HTTExonQ25-injected WT and R6/2 mice except for intrasession habituation at 4 weeks of age. Given that this difference was present only at 4-weeks and that this affect did not extend to activity change ratio at this time point, it appears to be more consistent with an exacerbated immune response to the presence of BSA than to a beneficial effect of Q25 on short-term memory performance. This is supported by previously published reports of the immunogenic properties of bovine serum albumin to the developing mouse brain (Habicht and Terres, 1966). The fact that cognitive tests at 4-weeks of age were most impacted is also consistent with this interpretation as it matches the pattern of behavioral abnormalities observed one month after injection of LPS, which is well-known to induce acute neuroinflammation (Sorrenti et al., 2018). To support this hypothesis we counted the number of microglia present around the site of injection 1 hr post-surgery. At this time point, we did not observe any difference in immune activation between groups. This does not necessarily exclude an immune response as LPS-induced inflammatory effects even *in vitro* require more than 1 hr to reach a maximal effect (Chae et al., 2017) and *in vivo* experiments generally focus on 24 hrs post-injection (Sorrenti et al., 2018; Zhao et al., 2017) although changes in Iba-1 expression have been observed as early as 2 hrs (Sorrenti et al., 2018). Given the focus on later time points with the very immunogenic nature of LPS, it is not surprising that an immune response is not observed 1 hr post-injection.

Aside from supporting a detrimental effect of HTTExon1Q48, this experiment also highlighted the importance of the age of animals at the time of injection. The ventricular injection site, injection volume (bilateral 2 µg injection vs. unilateral 2 µg injection) and age led to a much more rapid onset of phenotype in the R6/2 paradigm with more apparent aggregation of WT huntingtin than in the adult WT paradigm. At 12 weeks of age, changes in behavior and endogenous HTT state were present in WT injected pups that did not arise until 12 or 16 months of age in injected adult WT and aggregation of WT HTT was observed in both R6/2 and WT mice, which was not observed at any time point in adult WT mice. This raises interesting questions regarding both the role of HTT in development as well as the role of development in prion protein spreading, in general. The increased concentration of fibrils may also have played a role, but it is unlikely that the two-fold increase when coupled with a change in site of injection could explain the 9-month difference in induction time that was observed between the two experiments.

To determine if central administration of fibrils is necessary to induce behavioral changes, WT mice received intravenous injection of fibrils. With this paradigm, no changes in behavior were observed at 3 months of age. This time point is early to expect a behavioral phenotype but the experiment was aborted because assessment of the blood revealed that peripheral infusion of HTT and mHTT fibrils resulted in an immune response. Interestingly, fibrillar HTTExon1Q48 induced the highest immune response that most probably effectively blocked exogenous fibrillar HTTExon1-mediated changes within the central nervous system.

The multiple models utilized in this study allows us to conclusively show that HTTExon1Q48 fibrils are taken up by cells, both *in vitro* and *in vivo*, and trigger cellular dysfunction and behavioral changes in cells and mice after uptake. These changes are also associated with changes in the state of endogenous HTT. Together, these results strongly suggest that at least certain forms of HTT are capable of spreading and seeding disease; in other words, HTT fibrils have prion-like properties. While the importance of prion-like spreading of mHTT within normal HD pathophysiology is still unknown, studies of healthy tissue grafts implanted into the brains of HD patients demonstrated that mHTT protein could be found in the grafted tissue originating from healthy individuals (Cicchetti et al., 2014). This grafted tissue was derived from healthy donors expressing HTT with non-pathogenic CAG expansions. Thus, the only possible source of mHTT was the surrounding tissue. These findings, together with our observations in R6/2 mice, suggest that spread may occur in the patients' central nervous system, thus contributing to disease progression. There is a large degree of heterogeneity in the clinical features of HD (Phillips et al., 2008) in patients with the same CAG repeat length, which implies that there are, as of yet, undescribed factors contributing to clinical presentation (Gusella et al., 1983). While these factors may have a genetic basis (e.g. tau and cognitive decline (Vuono et al., 2015), proteostasis and age of onset (Genetic Modifiers of Huntington's Disease (GeM-HD) Consortium, 2015; Kuiper et al., 2017) our data indicates that non-cell autonomous spread of mHTT is a novel modifier of HD disease progression.

1.7 Acknowledgements

This study was funded by the Canadian Institutes of Health Research (CIHR) to FC who is also recipient of a Researcher Chair from the Fonds de recherche du Québec (FRQS) en santé providing salary support and operating funds. GS and AM are supported by FRQS doctoral research awards. AM is additionally supported by an O'Brien Foundation Fellowship. HLD is supported by a Desjardins scholarship from the Fondation du CHU de Québec and a bourse d'excellence du Centre Thématique de Recherche en Neurosciences (CTRN) du CHU de Québec. FL was supported by a Joseph Demers scholarship award from Université Laval. MA is supported by a post-doctoral fellowship from FRQS. RM and LB are supported by CNRS.

1.8 Contribution

MM carried out most of the *in vitro* and post-mortem analyses, and I contributed to writing the manuscript.

G.S. performed behavioral tests and analyses.

A.M. performed behavioral tests and analyses.

L.B. produced the material (synthetic fibrils) used in all experiments.

H.D. was involved in analyses and in assembling all figures.

F.L. carried out some *in vitro* experiments and analyses (percentage of contribution: 10%).

L.D. contributed to the intellectual design and some experimental approaches.

M.S-P. provided technical support for some experiments.

J.H.K. contributed intellectually to the development of the study design and experimental approaches. He provided material necessary for the experimental setup and reviewed the manuscript.

R.M. contributed intellectually to the overall study design and experimental approaches. He provided the material necessary and reviewed the manuscript.

M.A. participated in troubleshooting experimental problems, assisted in designing experiments and suggesting experimental approaches and helped image *in vivo* and *in vitro* work. She also wrote the first full draft of the manuscript.

F.C. was responsible for initial study design, experimental design and interpretation and analysis of data. She reviewed and corrected the first draft of the manuscript.

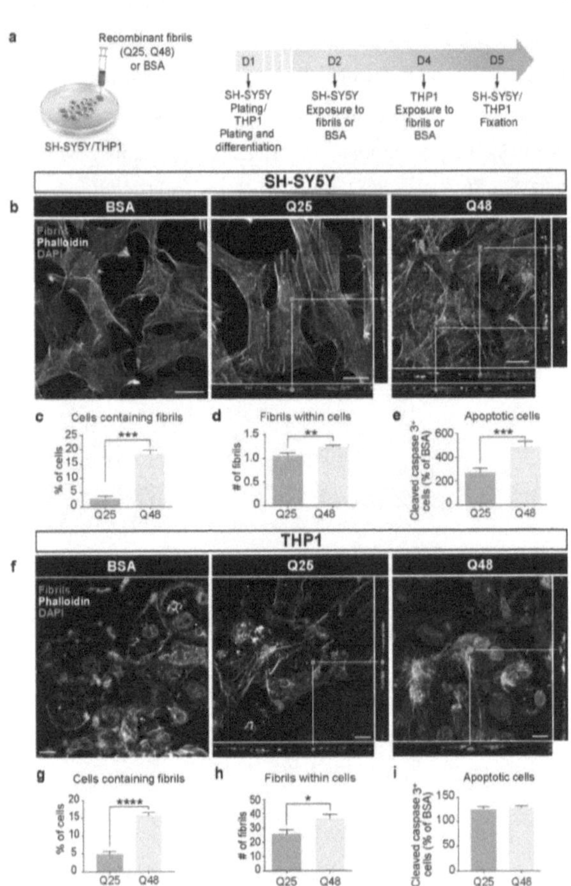

Figure 1.1. Uptake of fibrillar HTTExon1Q25 and Q48 by different cell types. Schematic of experimental design (**a**). Representative confocal photomicrographs of human SH-SY5Y cells (**b**) and THP1-derived macrophages (**f**) demonstrating uptake of both ATTO488-labeled HTTExon1Q25 and Q48 fibrils (green), 72 (SH-SY5Y) and 24 h (THP1) post-exposure, respectively. For all photomicrographs, the cell membrane was labelled with phalloidin (white) and cell nuclei were stained with DAPI (purple). The percentage of SH-SY5Y (**c**) and THP1 (**g**) cells containing puncta, the number of puncta per SH-SY5Y (**d**) and THP1 (**h**) cell and the number of apoptotic SH-SY5Y (**e**) and THP1 (**i**) cells were all calculated. All graphs are the average of three independent experiments. Data are expressed as mean ± SEM. Statistical analysis was performed using a students' unpaired t test. *p < 0.05, **p < 0.01, ***p < 0.001, ****p < 0.0001. Scale bars b = 25 μm, f = 10 μm. BSA bovine serum albumin, D day.

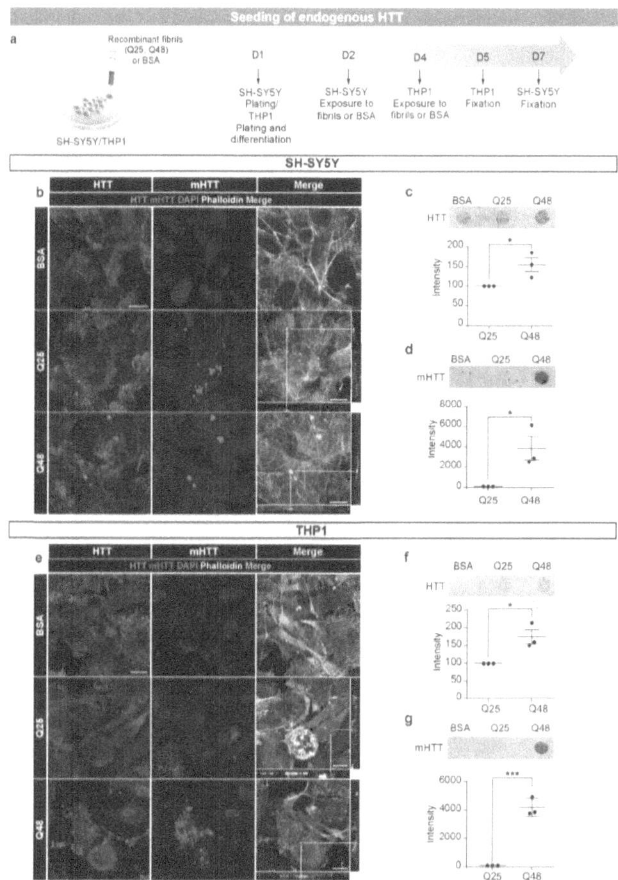

Figure 1.2. Seeding of endogenous HTT by exogenous HTTExon1Q48 fibrils. Schematic of experimental design for SH-SY5Y cells and THP1-derived macrophages (**a**). Representative confocal photomicrographs of cells exposed to ATTO550-labeled HTTExon1Q25/Q48 fibrils for 5 days (SH-SY5Y—**b**) and 24 h (THP1—**e**). Filter retardation assay and quantification of HTT aggregation immunodetected with anti-WT HTT antibody MAB2166 and anti-aggregated HTT antibody EM48 for SH-SY5Y (**c, d**) and THP1 (**f, g**) cells. For all filter retardation assay quantifications, the Q48 intensity is shown as percentage of the intensity of Q25. For immunofluorescence, endogenous HTT was detected with MAB2170 (green), HTTExon1Q25 and Q48 (red) and cell nuclei were stained with DAPI (blue). All graphs are the average of three independent experiments. Data are expressed as mean ± SEM. Statistical analysis was performed using a students' unpaired t test (**f**). *p < 0.05, ***p < 0.001. Scale bars = 10 μm. BSA bovine serum albumin, D day, GFP green fluorescent protein, HTT huntingtin, mHTT mutant huntingtin.

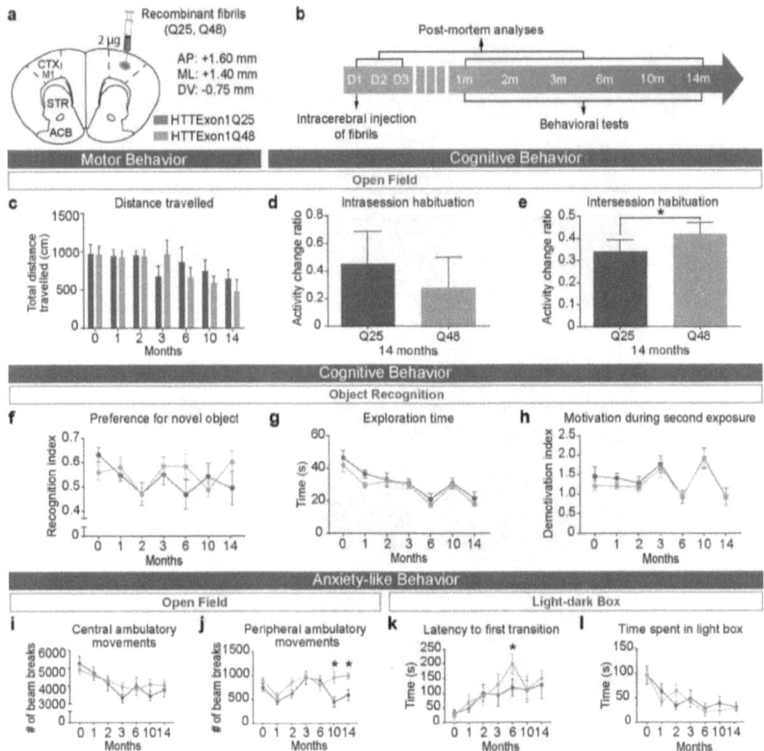

Figure 1.3. Manifestation of behavioral impairments in adult WT mice injected with HTTExon1Q48 fibrils. Atlas coordinates for intracerebral injections, treatment legend (**a**) and experimental timeline (**b**). Animals underwent motor, cognitive and anxiety-like behavioral tests from 1 to 14 months post-injection. Motor behavior was assessed using total distance traveled in 60 min in the open field (**c**). At 14 months post-injection, short-term memory was evaluated by assessing the change in distance traveled between the first 5 and the last 5 min of testing (**d**) and long-term memory was assessed by calculating the change in distance traveled in the first 5 min of baseline to 14 months post-injection (**e**). Cognitive performance was assessed at each time point by measuring the preference for the novel object (**f**). The absence of confounding factors was determined by measuring the exploration time (**g**) and motivation during the exposure to the novel object (**h**). Anxiety-like behavior was assessed in the open field by quantifying the distance traveled in the center of the open field (**i**) and in the periphery (**j**) as well as in the light–dark box by latency to leave the dark box (**k**) and total time spent in the light box (**l**). Data are expressed as mean ± SEM. Baseline HTTExon1Q25 n = 12, HTTExon1Q48 n = 12; 1 month HTTExon1Q25 n = 11, HTTExon1Q48 n = 11; 2 months HTTExon1Q25 n = 10, HTTExon1Q48 n = 10; 3–14 months HTTExon1Q25 n = 9, HTTExon1Q48 n = 9. Statistical analysis was performed using a students' unpaired t test for individual time points and a two-way ANOVA followed by Tukey's post hoc test for across time graphs. *p < 0.05. ACB nucleus accumbens, AP antero-posterior, CTX M1 primary motor cortex, D day, DV dorso-ventral, m month, ML medio-lateral, s seconds, STR striatum.

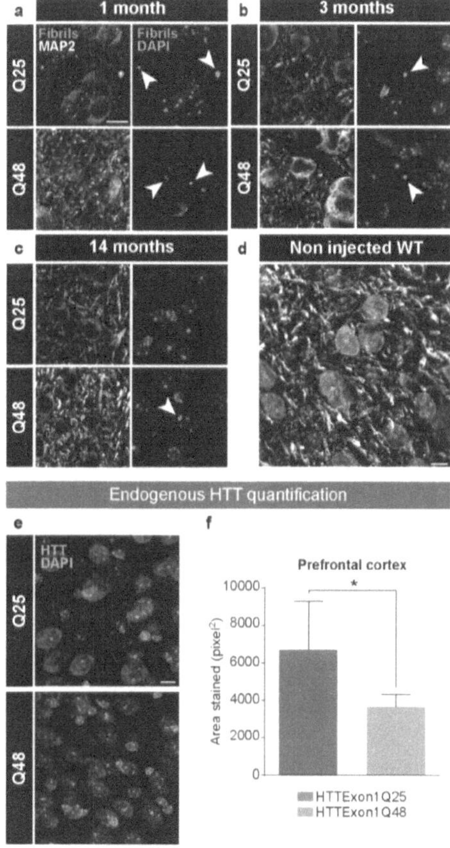

Figure 1.4. Post-mortem identification of HTTExon1Q25 and Q48 fibrils in adult WT mice. Representative confocal photomicrographs of brain tissue of WT mice sacrificed 1 month (HTTExon1Q25 n = 2, HTTExon1Q48 n = 2) (**a**), 3 months (HTTExon1Q25 n = 2, HTTExon1Q48 n = 2) (**b**), and 14 months (HTTExon1Q25 n = 8, HTTExon1Q48 n = 8) (**c**) post-injection and immunostained for HTTExon1 (green) and MAP2 (white). Arrowheads indicate the localization of fibrils. Specificity of anti-HTTExon1 antibody was assessed by staining a non-injected WT mouse (**d**). Representative confocal photomicrographs of brain tissue of WT sacrificed at 14 months post-surgery and immunostained for endogenous HTT (orange) (**e**). Quantification of HTT intensity as measured by total area stained in the prefrontal cortex (**f**). Nuclei were detected with DAPI (purple **a–d**; blue **e**). Data are expressed as mean ± SEM. WT Q25 n = 7, WT Q48 n = 7. Statistical analysis was performed using a students' unpaired t test. *p < 0.05. Scale bars = 10 μm. HTT huntingtin, MAP2 microtubule-associated protein 2, WT wild-type. Arrowheads indicate the localization of fibrils.

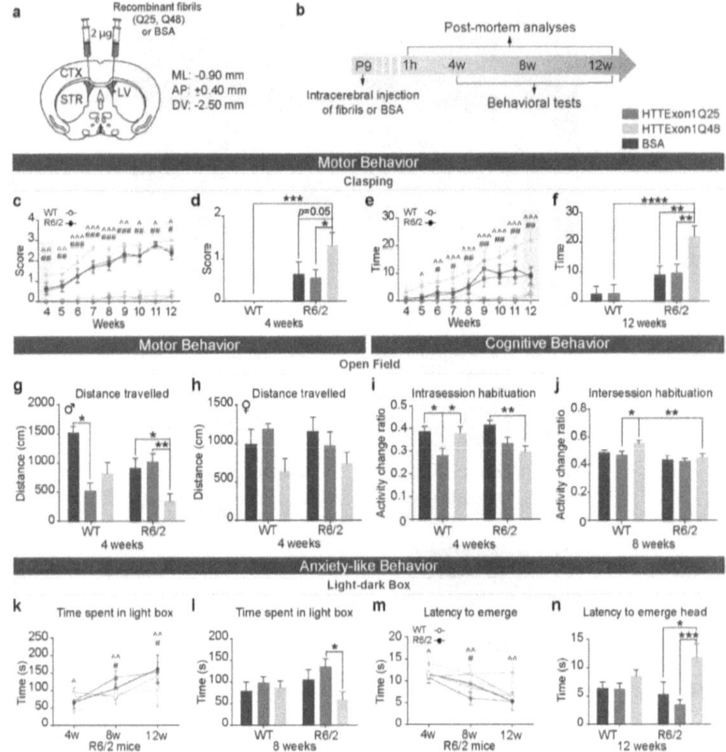

Figure 1.5. Precipitation of behavioral phenotype in R6/2 mice following injection of HTTExon1Q48 fibrils. Atlas coordinates for intraventricular injections, treatment legend (**a**) and experimental timeline (**b**). Clasping score in R6/2 mice at all tested time points (**c**) and at 4 weeks of age (**d**). Duration of full-clasping behavior at all tested time points (**e**) and at 12 weeks of age (**f**) WT BSA n = 13–14; WT HTTExon1Q25 n = 11–13; WT HTTExon1Q48 n = 12–15; R6/2 BSA n = 11–14; R6/2 HTTExon1Q25 n = 12–18; R6/2 HTTExon1Q48 n = 9–19. Motor endurance was measured by assessing the distance traveled in the last 5 min of the open field at 4 weeks post-injection for male (**g**) and female mice (**h**). WT BSA n = 9F, 4M; WT HTTExon1Q25 n = 3F, 10M; WT HTTExon1Q48 n = 8F, 9M; R6/2 BSA n = 7F, 9M; R6/2 HTTExon1Q25 n = 7F, 10M; R6/2 HTTExon1Q48 n = 11F, 8M. At 4 weeks post-injection, short-term memory was evaluated by assessing the change in distance traveled between the first 5 min and min 25–30 of testing (**i**) and at 8 weeks post-injection, long-term memory was measured by calculating the change in distance traveled between the first 10 min of testing at 4 and 8 weeks post-injection (**j**). WT BSA n = 12–13; WT HTTExon1Q25 n = 12–13; WT HTTExon1Q48 n = 14–15; R6/2 BSA n = 12–16 R6/2 HTTExon1Q25 n = 16–17; R6/2Q HTTExon148 n = 16–19. Anxietylike behavior was assessed in the light–dark box using time spent in the light box at 4, 8 and 12 weeks of age (**k**) and at 8 weeks only (**l**) and latency to emerge head at 4, 8 and 12 weeks of age (**m**) and at 12 weeks only (**n**). WT HTTExon1Q25 n = 11–14; WT HTTExon1Q48 n = 11–17; R6/2 HTTExon1Q25 n = 8–14; R6/2 HTTExon1Q48 n = 8–17. Data are expressed as mean ± SEM. For c, i, k, and m, statistics were calculated using a linear mixed effects model. For all other graphs, statistics were performed using a two-way ANOVA with Tukey's post hoc test. *p < 0.05, **p < 0.01. AP antero-posterior, CTX cortex, DV dorso-ventral, F female h hour, LV lateral ventricle, M male, ML medio-lateral, s seconds, P9 post-natal day 9, STR striatum, w weeks, WT wild-type.

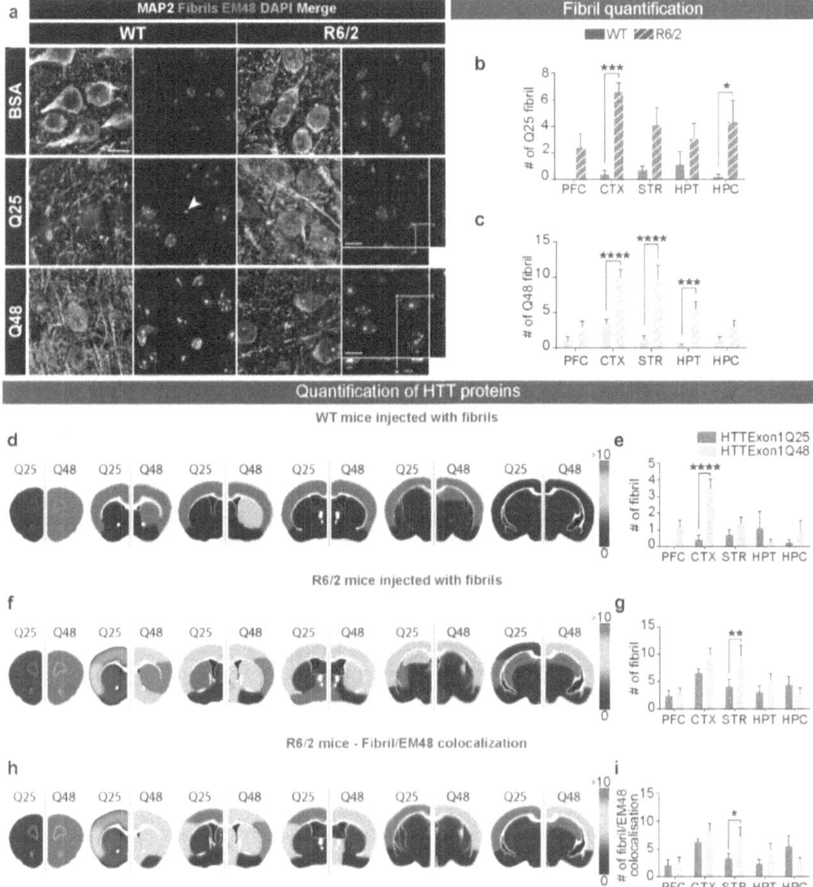

Figure 1.6. Colocalization of HTTExon1Q48 fibrils and endogenous mHTT in R6/2 mice. Representative confocal photomicrographs of fibrils in the brains of WT and R6/2 mice at 12 weeks post-injection (**a**). Arrowheads indicate the localization of fibrils. BSA-injected mice were used as negative controls to set the lasers on the confocal microscope. Direct comparison of puncta number between WT and R6/2 mice injected HTTExon1Q25 (**b**) and HTTExon1Q48 (**c**). Heat maps depicting the number of puncta detected in different brain regions by converting low numbers of puncta to dark blue, and high numbers to red, in WT (**d**) and R6/2 mice (**f**). The corresponding graphs are displayed for WT (**e**) and R6/2 mice (**g**). The colocalization between EM48 and HTT fibrils depicted as a heat map (**h**) and graph (**i**). Quadruple immunofluorescence of injected fibrils (green), endogenous aggregates EM48 (red), microtubule-associated protein MAP2 (white) and cell nuclei DAPI (purple). Scale bars = 10 μm. Data are expressed as mean ± SEM. WT HTTExon1Q25 n = 5, WT HTTExon1Q48 n = 5, R6/2 HTTExon1Q25 n = 5, R6/2 HTTExon1Q48 n = 5. Statistics are performed using a two-way ANOVA with Tukey's post hoc tests. *p < 0.05, **p < 0.01, ***p < 0.001, ****p < 0.0001. BSA bovine serum albumin, CTX cortex, HPC hippocampus, HPT hypothalamus, MAP2 microtubule-associated protein 2, PFC, prefrontal cortex, STR striatum, WT wild-type.

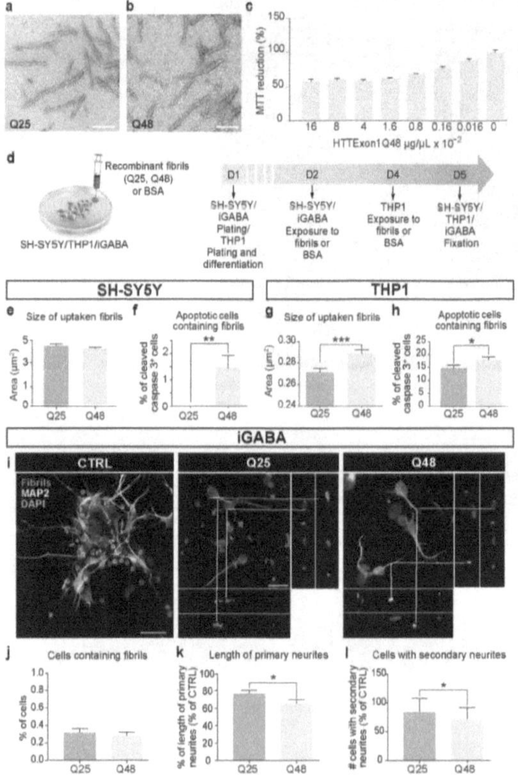

Figure 1.7. Toxic effects of exogenous HTTExon1Q48 fibrils on multiple cell lines. Representative electron microscopy images of HTTExon1Q25 (**a**) and Q48 fibrils (**b**). Dose response curve showing reduction in MTT levels after exposure to increasing concentrations of HTTExon1Q48 fibrils (**c**). Experimental design and timeline of treatment with ATTO488-labeled HTTExon1Q25 and Q48 fibrils (**d**). The size of HTTExon1Q25 and 48 fibrils within SH-SY5Y (**e**) and THP1 cells (**g**) were measured. The population of cells containing fibrils was isolated and within this population, an increase in the percentage of caspase 3+ cells was detected in both SH-SY5Y (**f**) and THP1 (**h**) cells after exposure to HTTExon1Q48 fibrils. In THP1 cells, the size of intracellular aggregates (**g**) and the number of caspase 3+ cells containing fibrils (**h**) were also quantified. The percentage of caspase 3+ cells in HTTExon1Q25 and HTTExon1Q48 cells was calculated compared to BSA control (**h**). iGABA neurons demonstrate uptake of both HTTExon1Q25 and HTTExon1Q48 fibrils after treatment. Immunostaining against microtubule-associated protein MAP2 (white) and DAPI staining to mark the nuclei (blue) were performed, while fibrils labeled with ATTO-488 (**i**). The number of cells with puncta were counted (**j**). The effect of fibrils on morphology was assessed by measuring the length each cell's primary neurite (**k**) and the number of neurons with secondary projections (**l**). Scale bars **a and b** = 100 nm; **i** = 10 μm. Data are expressed as mean +/- SEM. Statistical analysis was performed using student's unpaired t-test. All graphs are the average of three independent replicates. *p<0.05, ** p<0.01. BSA bovine serum albumin, CTRL control, D day, MAP2 microtubule-associated protein 2.

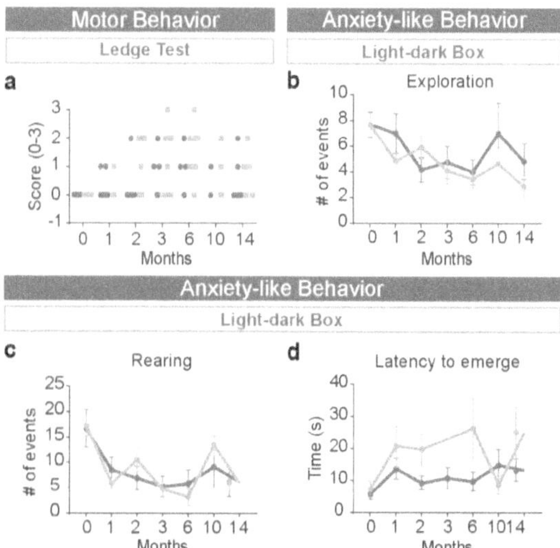

Figure 1.8. Absence of motor impairments in WT adult mice injected with HTTExon1Q48 fibrils. Motor performance was characterized using the ledge test (**a**). Motor confound were absent from the light-dark box as measured by exploration (**b**) and rearing (**c**). Anxiety-like behavior by analysis of latency to emerge head from the dark box in the light-dark box test (**d**). Data are expressed as mean +/- SEM. HttExon1Q25 n=9-12, HTTExon1Q48 n=9-12. Statistical analysis was calculated using a repeated measures two-way ANOVA with Tukey's post-hoc tests. S seconds.

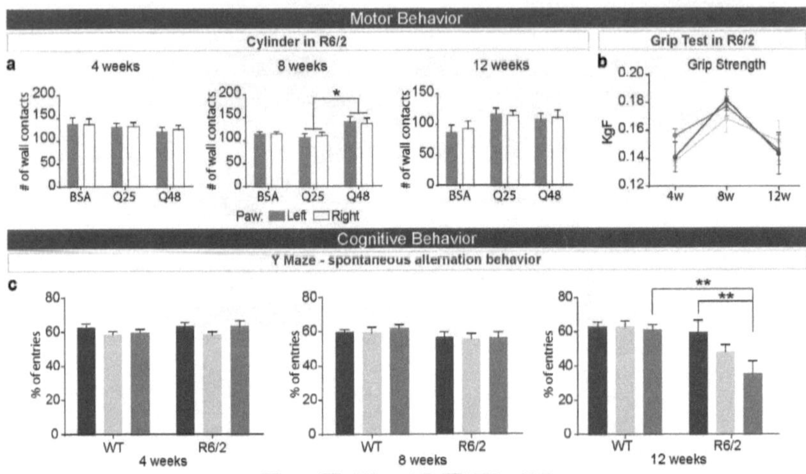

Figure 1.9. **Examples of behavioral measures not affected in R6/2 mice following injection of HTTExon1Q48 fibrils.** Motor performance in R6/2 mice was also assessed using the cylinder task (R6/2 BSA n=9-16; R6/2 HTTExon1Q25 n=12-17; R6/2 HTTExon1Q48 n=9-18) (**a**) and grip test (R6/2 BSA n=9; R6/2 HTTExon1Q25 n=13; R6/2 HTTExon1Q48 n=9) (**b**). Cognitive performance was measured at 4, 8 and 12 weeks of age using the Y-maze (WT BSA n=12-13; WT HTTExon1Q25 n=10-13; WT HTTExon1Q48 n=10-14; R6/2 BSA n=8-16; R6/2 HTTExon1Q25 n=12-15; R6/2 HTTExon1Q48 n=9-18) (**c**). Data are expressed as mean +/- SEM. Statistical analysis was performed using a two-way ANOVA with Tukey's post-hoc tests except for **b** where a repeated measures two-way ANOVA was performed. *p<0.05. BSA bovine serum albumin, w, weeks, WT wild-type.

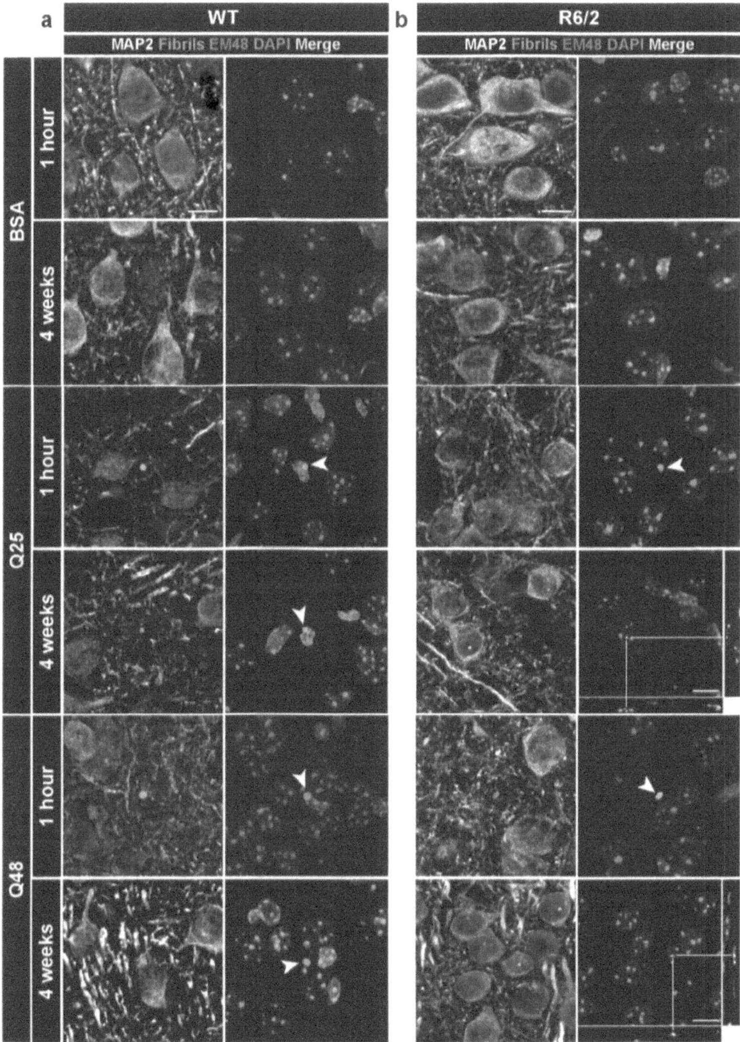

Figure 1.10. Colocalization of HTTExon1Q48 fibrils with endogenous mHTT in R6/2 mice at 4 weeks of age. Fibrillar puncta were detected in WT (a) and R6/2 mice brains (b) at 1 h and 4 weeks post-injection of HTTExon1Q25 and Q48, but not BSA. Arrowheads indicate puncta. Quadruple immunofluorescence for fibrils (green), mHTT aggregates EM48 (red), MAP2 (white) and cell nuclei DAPI (purple). Merged EM48 and fibrillar puncta is visualized with yellow. Scale bars: 10 μm. BSA bovine serum albumin MAP2 microtubule-associated protein 2, WT wild-type.

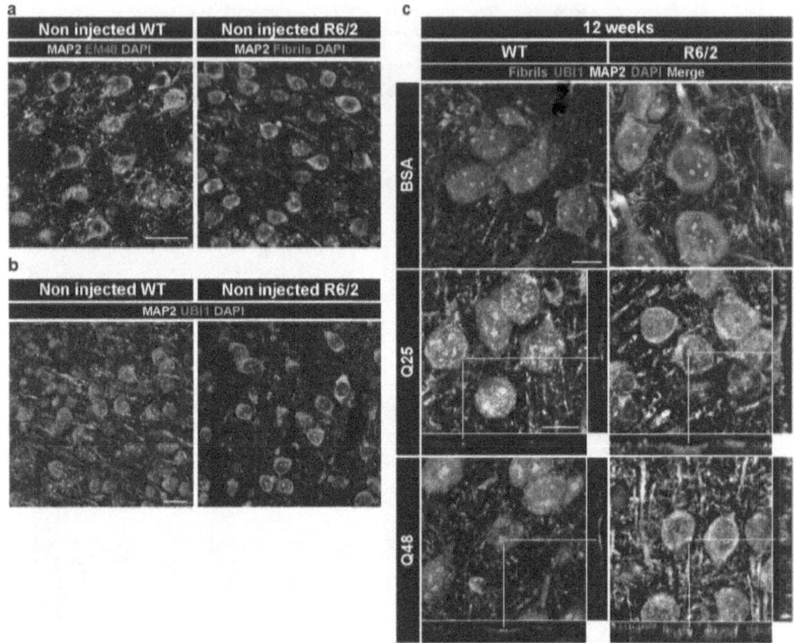

Figure 1.11. Colocalization of HTTExon1Q48 fibrils with ubiquitin. The specificity of EM48 (**a**) and ubiquitin (UBI1) (**b**) was confirmed in non injected WT and R6/2 mice. To further support this, UBI1 staining was used as an additional marker of endogenous mHTT. It did not colocalize with fibrils in WT mice, but in R6/2 mice (**c**), particularly R6/2 mice injected with HTTExon1Q48 fibrils at 12 weeks post-injection. Quadruple immunofluorescence for fibrils (green), mHTT aggregates by either ubiquitin or EM48 (red), MAP2 (white) and cell nuclei DAPI (purple/blue). Scale bar **a, b** = 10 µm; **c**= 20 µm. MAP2 microtubule-associated protein 2, WT wild-type.

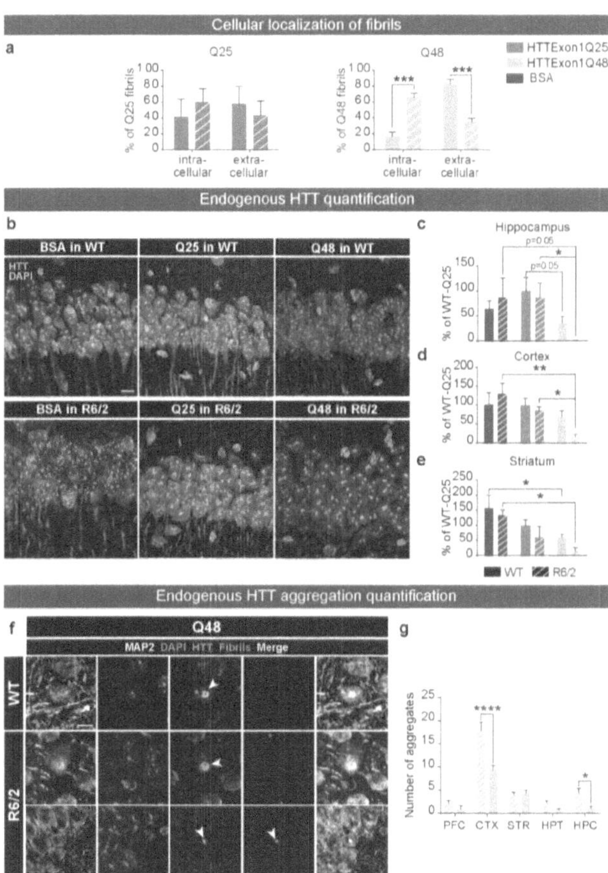

Figure 1.12. Changes in staining patterns of endogenous HTT following injection of HTTExon1Q48 fibrils. The presence of fibrillar puncta inside and outside the cells was quantified for HTTExon1Q25 and Q48 fibrils in WT and R6/2 mice (**a**). WT HTTExon1Q25 n=5, WT HTTExon1Q48 n=5, R6/2 HTTExon1Q25 n=5, R6/2 HTTExon1Q48 n=5. Representative confocal photomicrographs of endogenous HTT immunoreactivity in the hippocampus of WT and R6/2 mice (**b**) and quantification of staining intensity for hippocampus (**c**), cortex (**d**) and striatum (**e**). Quantification data is shown as percentage of area stained for Q25-treated WT controls. WT BSA n=5; WT HTTExon1Q25 n=6; WT HTTExon1Q48 n=6, R6/2 BSA n=3, R6/2 HTTExon1Q25 n=2-4, R6/2 HTTExon1Q48 n=6. Representative confocal photomicrographs depicting changes in the staining pattern of endogenous HTT in the animals injected with Q48 (**f**) and quantification of the number of endogenous HTT aggregates detected in different brain regions (**g**). WT HTTExon1Q25 n=10, WT HTTExon1Q48 n=10, R6/2 HTTExon1Q25 n=10, R6/2 HTTExon1Q48 n=10. Data are expressed as mean +/- SEM. Statistical analysis was performed using a two-way ANOVA with Tukey's post-hoc tests. *p<0.05, *** p<0.001. Scale bar = 10 µm. BSA bovine serum albumin, CTX cortex, HPC hippocampus, HPT hypothalamus, HTT huntingtin, MAP2 microtubule-associated protein 2, PFC, prefrontal cortex, STR striatum, WT wild-type.

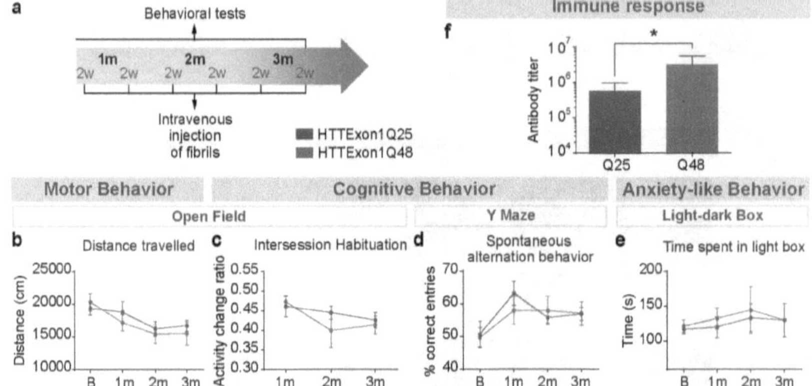

Figure 1.13. Development of an immune response following intravenous injection of HTTExon1Q25 and Q48 fibrils in adult WT mice. Experimental timeline (**a**). Motor performance was assessed using distance travelled in the first 5 min in the open field (**b**). Long-term memory was measured by the change in distance travelled in the first 5 min of each testing time point (**c**). Working memory was measured by spontaneous alternations in the Y-maze (**d**). Anxiety-like behavior was measured by time spent in the light box of the light-dark box (**e**). Blood was collected at the end of the experiment and the antibody titre in HTTExon1Q25 and Q48 injected mice was assessed (**f**). Data are expressed as mean +/- SEM. WT HTTExon1Q25 n=8, WT HTTExon1Q48 n=7. Statistical analysis was performed using a repeated measures two-way ANOVA with Tukey's post-hoc tests except for **f** where a student's unpaired t-test was utilized. *p<0.05. B baseline, BSA bovine serum albumin, m month, s seconds, w week, WT wild-type.

Conclusions and perspectives

In the following sections, I will discuss our observations, what I believe they have contributed to the field, technical considerations and limitations of the study as well as some of the future perspectives.

2.1 Results

My Ph.D. book builds on the initial observations reported by Dr. Cicchetti and her co-workers (Cicchetti et al., 2014; Jeon et al., 2016) that mHTT may behave in a prion-like manner. Although these studies showed mHTT spreading in *in vitro* and *in vivo* paradigms (Jeon et al., 2016), they did not disclose the exact mechanisms underlying its propagation, nor if extracellular mHTT could, once uptaken, corrupt endogenous HTT. Recent literature has suggested that mHTT can propagate via synaptic connections, TNTs, exosomes or by breaching the plasma membrane with active or passive transport (Masnata and Cicchetti, 2017). Once inside the cell, mHTT has a high affinity to bind lipidic membranes of cellular organelles, disrupting or altering their functionality (Kegel et al., 2009, 2000; Ren et al., 2009). It has also been reported that mHTT recruits WT HTT and triggers a seeding process (Ren et al., 2009; Ruiz-Arlandis et al., 2016; Trevino et al., 2012). To shed light on this, we selected fibrillar exon 1 fragment of the human mHTT protein - which has already been shown to propagate between cellular elements and recruit endogenous HTT in cell culture systems (Pieri et al., 2012; Ren et al., 2009) - and introduced them to different cells and animal models.

The work Masnata et al. provided evidence for the capacity of mHTT to spread and seed disease in multiple *in vitro* and *in vivo* settings. We showed how HTTExon1 fibrils with expanded polyQ repeats could be uptaken by different cells in *in vitro* conditions and provoked detrimental effects. For example, uptake induced apoptosis and the recruitment of endogenous HTT in both cultured neuronal-like cells and macrophages, while it also negatively impacted dendrites of cultured GABAergic neurons. When injected intracerebrally into WT adult mice, HTTExon1Q48 fibrils triggered a cognitive and anxiety-like behavior, spread to surrounding areas and modified the staining pattern of endogenous

HTT. Additionally, the intraventricular administration of HTTExon1Q48 fibrils in R6/2 mice exacerbated and precipitated motor and cognitive deficits, spread from the lateral ventricles to distal cerebral areas, colocalized with endogenous mHTT aggregates and disrupted normal HTT staining patterns. Finally, we observed that the injection of HTTExon1Q48 fibrils directly into the bloodstream of WT mice gave rise to an immune response.

2.2 Contribution to the field

The misfolding and aggregation of proteins is a typical hallmark of several proteinopathies, including neurodegenerative disorders such as AD, PD, HD and prion diseases (Soto and Pritzkow, 2018) although the latter, are extremely rare and the only ones considered infectious (Prusiner, 1982). In prion diseases, the normal prion protein adopts an abnormal conformation, which is in turn capable of seeding disease independently. This consequently triggers an exponential amplification of the pathological prion. In this fashion, the abnormally misfolded prion rapidly spreads across the CNS and can infect individuals of the same, or different species (Prusiner, 1982). Prion diseases such as CJD progress rapidly and death occurs within 1 year of onset. While AD, PD and HD are not classified as infectious diseases, their causative pathological proteins share analogies with the prion (Prusiner, 2012).

Release and uptake mechanisms are thought to confer a more or less infectious asset to the various prion-like proteins. mHTT, tau, α-syn and Aβ have all been shown to propagate transsynaptically (Clavaguera et al., 2009; Luk et al., 2012a; Meyer-Luehmann et al., 2006; Pecho-Vrieseling et al., 2014; Walker et al., 2002), however, inoculation of these proteins in different experimental conditions (**Table 4 and 5**) reveals distinct propagating efficiency, where mHTT is seemingly less prone to spreading. Interestingly, the axonal transport is thought to influence the transsynaptic propagation. While mHTT fibrils are transported uniquely retrogradely, α-syn and Aβ42 fibrils are transported both retrogradely and anterogradely. Following an anterograde transport, both α-syn and Aβ42 fibrils are released at the synaptic terminal (Brahic et al., 2016). The absence of mHTT anterograde transport may be associated with the lower incidence of synaptic propagation.

The propagation of prion-like proteins such as tau, α-syn and mHTT is also facilitated by the TNTs. TNTs allow direct communication between cells. They are generated in homeostatic conditions but also under specific stimuli. For instance, intracellular overexpression of mHTT induces TNTs formation, resulting in mHTT transport from cell to cell (Costanzo et al., 2013). Similarly, the cells respond to an excess of α-syn aggregates forming TNTs and transferring α-syn-containing lysosomes to acceptor cells (Saida Abounit et al., 2016). Extracellular signaling can also promote TNTs synthesis. In fact, extracellular propagating tau can activate the formation of TNTs and subsequently promote transneuronal spreading (Tardivel et al., 2016). This suggests that pathological protein expression is linked to biological stimuli that induce TNTs formation and consequent protein spreading.

T-cell infiltration and activation of microglia into the brain are predominant in neurodegenerative diseases. These immune cells may play a role in the propagation of prion-like proteins. For instance, hyperstimulation of microglia provokes α-syn aggregation and promotes the transfer of pathological α-syn seed in the CNS (George et al., 2019). Analogously, the activation of microglia is linked to tau hyperphosphorylation and propagation (Španić et al., 2019). In contrast, the overexpression of mHTT within microglia induces a cell-autonomous transcriptional activation enhancing an inflammatory response subsequently leading to neuronal death (Crotti et al., 2014). Under these circumstances, necrotic cells may release mHTT that would be free to propagate to neighboring cells. As of today, it appears that the immune system might dictate the progression of neurodegenerative diseases also directly or indirectly contributing to prion-like propagation.

Once proteins are released in the extracellular space, they can either be degraded or taken up by other cells. It has been described that both mHTT and α-syn, possibly by their capacity to interact with the lipids of the plasma membrane (Pieri et al., 2012), can reach the intracellular compartment by passive transport (Ren et al., 2009). Additionally, both fibrils can be actively internalized via clathrin-dependent endocytosis (Oh et al., 2016; Ruiz-Arlandis et al., 2016) and α-syn fibrils alone can also be transported by HSPGs-binding (Holmes et al., 2013). Molecular charges and weight, protein structure and selective cell-surface receptors are therefore directly implicated in protein propagation efficiency.

In comparison to other proteins, the prion-like behavior of mHTT is not as well established. Masnata et al. and follow-up studies were conducted to provide a better insight into the spreading and seeding capacities of mHTT and how this contributes to the development of HD (**Table 5**). In particular, these studies aimed to unravel the routes and extent of mHTT spreading, as well as to analyze the behavioral and neuropathological outcomes of such events. A good proportion of the work performed by Dr. Cicchetti's lab aimed to validate the transneuronal propagation of mHTT, injecting different mHTT inocula (HD and JHD brain homogenates, mHTTExon1 synthetic fibrils, and HTTExon1Q103 transduced via AAV2/6) into the cortex of WT animals. However, these studies did not lead to significant mHTT propagation, but instead showed that the spread was restricted to areas in close proximity to the injection site and accompanied by transient or mild HD-like neuropathology (Gosset et al., 2020; Masnata et al., 2019; Maxan et al., 2020).

This inconsistency can be explained by the differences of inoculum, injection site and experimental time points used in these studies. For instance, it has previously been reported that full-length mHTT contained into human HD fibroblasts, iPSCs and derived exosomes can propagate across distant cerebral regions and induce HD-like behavioral and pathophysiological features in WT mice (Jeon et al., 2016). In contrast, HTTExon1 fragments, either expressed by a viral transduction (Maxan et al., 2020) or artificially assembled and injected in the cerebral tissue (Masnata et al, 2019), failed to reproduce the extent of similar events (Masnata et al., 2019; Maxan et al., 2020). This may suggest that the full-length mHTT spreads more aggressively. However, it should be noted that those inocula contained full-length mHTT with a polyQ length equal to 143. Given that the polyQ length among HD patients averages 42-43 (Capiluppi et al., 2020) and that, generally, CAG length correlates with disease severity and age of onset (e.g. JHD) (Langbehn et al., 2010), we could speculate that the polyQ length contributes to disease spread and seed at which this occurs. A study conducted in drosophila supports this hypothesis since HTTExon1Q138 efficiently spread from the olfactory receptor neurons, where it was expressed, to the distant but synaptically connected large posterior neurons (Babcock and Ganetzky, 2015). Similar phenomena are observed in studies with more complex organisms such as rats and mice (Ceccarelli et al., 2016; DiFiglia et al 2007; Franich et al., 2008; Pecho-Vrieseling et al.,

2016). In fact, the transduction of mHTTExon1 with extended polyQ in a targeted cerebral area (respectively Q138; Q100; Q70; Q72;) via AAV (Ceccarelli et al., 2016; DiFiglia et al 2007; Franich et al., 2008) or lentiviral vectors (Pecho-Vrieseling et al., 2016) induced a widespread diffusion of the viral-expressed mHTT.

When comparing the propagation and seeding capacity of two mHTT inocula with relatively similar polyQ expansions (human HD brain homogenate Q52 vs HTTExon1Q48 fibrils), we observed striking differences (Gosset et al., 2020; Masnata et al., 2019). Despite the use of similar experimental parameters (e.g. mHTT administration to both WT and transgenic mice, intracortical injections, administration in adult age, similar timeline and battery of behavioral tests), mHTT-derived from human homogenates showed less efficiency to propagate and failed to induce behavioral changes in WT mice, while it only triggered a mild phenotype in the BACHD model. The HD homogenates also did not induce any modification in staining patterns of endogenous HTT, which was observed in both WT and HD mice following HTTExon1Q48 fibrils (Gosset et al., 2020; Masnata et al., 2019). It can be hypothesized that the homogenization process and the presence of interfering solutes different from mHTT could have disrupted or dilute the concentration of spreading and seeding-competent mHTT. In contrast, the artificial synthesis of purified mHTT fibrils with similar polyQ repeats more closely mimics the mHTT prion-like behavior.

The age of exposure to extracellular mHTT can presumably play a role in promoting mHTT prion-like behavior. For instance, the injection into the lateral ventricles of neonatal mice is associated with mHTT propagation in distant cerebral areas in both WT and HD mice, which resulted in marked HD-like behavioral and neuropathological phenotypes (Jeon et al., 2016; Masnata et al., 2019). This could suggest that exposure to extracellular mHTT early in life can promote or accelerate disease development.

Although the vast majority of prior studies focused on mHTT propagation within the brain, mHTT is ubiquitously expressed throughout the human body, therefore discovering if peripheral mHTT, such as forms found in the plasma, could propagate to cerebral areas and induce pathology is also of interest. For example, injection of mHTT fibrils via the tail vein leads to an immune response that likely shields the CNS from mHTTExon1 fibrils-mediated changes (Masnata et al., 2019). Notably, the administration of fragments of prion-like proteins such as Aβ and tau was used to promote immunization as a therapeutic treatment. Exposure to Aβ and tau promoted a sustained expression of anti-Aβ and anti-tau antibodies in both preclinical and clinical studies (Alpaugh et al., 2019; Masnata et al., 2020). Following several years of clinical research, four anti-Aβ and two anti-tau vaccines are now tested in clinical trials for AD (Congdon and Sigurdsson, 2018; Schilling et al., 2018). For the field of immunotherapy, our finding could be a stepping stone to promote the study and application of active immunization as an HD therapeutic strategy.

A very elegant technique of parabiosis was also used to study peripheral mHTT propagation. This surgical procedure consists of anatomically joining two animals by their flank to induce vascular anastomoses. This methodology was initially used to investigate if blood from young mice possessed rejuvenation properties (Mccay et al., 1957). Subsequently, it was used to answer questions in fields related to blood circulation and inflammation (Abe et al., 2004; Donskoy and Goldschneider, 1992), tumor metastasis (Duyverman et al., 2012) and neurodegenerative diseases (Bu et al., 2018). A recent parabiosis study also described how the Aβ protein (Aβ) protein expressed by the APPswe/PS1dE9 transgenic AD mice propagated and accumulated in the brain of parabiotic WT mice. After 1 year of parabiosis, other AD hallmarks such as tau pathology, neuroinflammation and microhemorrhage were detected in the brains of the joined WT mouse, highlighting the toxicity of blood propagating Aβ (Bu et al., 2018). In Rieux et al. (Rieux et al., 2020), mHTT was found to propagate from the HD to the WT mouse through blood and was detected in several organs, including the liver, muscle, kidney and brain as early as 6 months post-surgery. Even though the parabiosis surgery impeded the performance of behavioral tests, the detrimental effects of mHTT were measured by vascular changes and HD pathological features found in the cortex of the WT parabiotic mice (Rieux et al., 2020). Notably, the joined bloodstream did not exclusively induce HD-like features in the otherwise healthy mouse, but it showed an improvement of various features associated with the CNS and periphery of the HD mouse (Rieux et al., 2020). These results highlight how the continuous supply of mHTT provided by the share bloodstream could be harmful to otherwise healthy organisms, and *vice versa*.

The potential recruitment of HTT by mHTT has been mostly investigated in *in vitro* systems, commonly artificially inducing the expression of various HTT and mHTT fragments (**Table**

3). For instance, the co-transfection of normal-length and extended polyQ in monkey-derived cells (Cos-1) demonstrated that the 2 polyQ ended up co-aggregating in a unique entity (Kazantsev et al., 1999; Busch et al., 2003). Cellular transfection of a large variety of human cells with HTTExon1Q25 and subsequent exposure to mHTT Q44 fibrils was also used to validate these findings (Ren et al., 2009; Trevino et al., 2012; Ruiz-Arlandis et al., 2016). In contrast, the work published by Dr. Cicchetti's lab illustrated the seeding of endogenous HTT by extracellular mHTT in 2 different human cell lines (SH-SY5Y and THP1 differentiated macrophages), showing an increase of mHTT SDS-insoluble aggregates. A decrease in the intensity of the normal HTT staining patterns was also detected in WT and R6/2 mice and non-human primates (Masnata et al., 2019; Maxan et al., 2020). The reduction of the staining pattern intensity could be interpreted as a change in WT HTT structural conformation or sequestration into aggregates. Notably, the observation of WT HTT-positive puncta in the brains of both WT and R6/2 mice might support the hypothesis of aggregate formation (Masnata et al., 2019). Alternatively, this decrease could be a sign of increased degradation or diminished protein transcription.

Several studies have now provided evidence for the mHTT prion-like capacity by showing that the administration of exogenous mHTT to either the CNS or periphery can induce HD-like changes or exacerbate HD-phenotype in WT and HD mice. This novel aspect of the disease will need to be taken into consideration when tailoring therapeutic approaches.

Inoculum	Injection site/administration site	Recipient/s	Outcome	Reference
Q138HTTExons 1–12	Olfactory receptor neurons	*Drosophila*	mHTT aggregates gathered at synaptic terminals and exponentially propagated throughout several brain regions	(Babcock and Ganetzky, 2015)
Lentivirus HTTExon1Q72	Cortex	WT adult mice	Transduced HTTExon1Q72 propagated neuron-to-neuron The mHTT propagation occurs throughout the cortical stratal pathway	(Pecho-Vrieseling et al., 2014)
AAV2/6 - HTTExon1Q103	Cortex	WT adult	Transient expression of motor and anxiety-like behavior Detection of mHTT within 3 months post injection	(Maxan et al., 2020)

			Limited mHTT propagation in the area surrounding the injection site Decreased endogenous HTT signal intensity	
	Putamen	Healthy non-human primates	Absence of HD-like behavior Detection of mHTT in the area surrounding the injection site	
HD patients derived fibroblasts (72, 143 and 180 CAG) iPSCs (143 CAG) Fibroblasts-derived exosomes	Lateral ventricles	WT neonatal mice	Detection of propagating mHTT within striatal neurons Development of motor disorders and cognitive impairments 3 months after injection (cells) and 4 weeks post injection (exosomes) Loss of DARPP32 positive neurons Striatal inflammation and gliosis Diffuse atrophy in the striatum	(Jeon et al., 2016)
Adult human HD brain homogenates	Cortex	WT adult mice	Unchanged behavior Propagation of exogenous mHTT from cortical injection sites to surrounding structures	(Gosset et al., 2020)
	Cortex	BACHD adult mice	Exacerbation of HD-like long-term memory abnormalities	
Human JHD brain homogenates	Putamen	Healthy non-human primates	Unaltered behavior Detection of exogenous mHTT within neurons 8 months post-injection	
Human synthetic HTTExon1Q48 fibrils	Cortex	WT adult mice	Development of anxiety-like and cognitive HD-phenotype respectively at 10- and 14-months post injection Detection of mHTT fibrils in the proximity of the injection site until 3 months post injection Altered endogenous HTT staining patter	(Masnata et al., 2019)
	Tail vein	WT adult mice	Clearance of mHTT fibrils by the host immune system	
	Lateral ventricles	R6/2 neonatal mice	Early induction and fast precipitation of motor, cognitive and anxiety-like behavior mHTT propagation throughout the brain Colocalization of mHTT fibrils with endogenous aggregates	

mHTT in zQ175 mouse blood	Blood circulation	WT adult mice	Altered endogenous HTT staining patter Diffusion of mHTT aggregates to CNS and periphery HD-like vascular pathology Decrease of markers of cell populations targeted in HD	(Rieux et al., 2020)

Table 5. *In vivo* **experimental evidence for the prion-like behavior of mHTT.**
Abbreviations: BACHD, Bacterial artificial chromosome (BAC) transgenic mouse model of HD; CNS, central nervous system; DARPP32, dopamine- and cAMP-regulated neuronal phosphoprotein; HD, Huntington's disease; HTT, huntingtin; iPSCs, Induced pluripotent stem cells mHTT, mutant huntingtin; Q, polyglutamine; WT, wild-type. Table made by Maria Masnata.

2.3 Technical considerations and limits

•   **The mHTT inoculum.** mHTT fibrils are just one of the multiple mHTT species that result from mHTT misfolding and aggregation. mHTT fibrils were chosen for this study because of their capacity to induce HD neuropathological features. However, other species, such as mHTT small monomers and oligomers, are known to spread and seed disease. A direct comparison of HTTExon1 fibrils with monomers and oligomers could have been more informative, possibly identifying which mHTT species would possess the most prominent prion-like capacities.

•   **The control inoculum.** In the *in vitro* experimental settings and in the treatment of the R6/2 and WT pups, BSA was used as a negative control. While for cell culture paradigms, this was a valuable and reliable negative control, in the animal study, BSA seemingly induced an immune response. Saline or blank injections could have been used as an alternative.

•   **Cell lines.** SH-SY5Y cell line is one of the most commonly used cell lines in neuroscience due to its human origin and the ability of the cells to differentiate into a catecholaminergic phenotype. This cell line has been extensively used in *in vitro* studies of mHTT fibrils uptake and interaction with the plasma membrane (Monsellier et al., 2016; Pieri et al., 2012; Ruiz-Arlandis et al., 2016). In our setup, however, we used undifferentiated SH-SY5Y cells, which scarcely express mature neuronal properties. Therefore, to complement the results obtained with the SH-SY5Y cells, we introduced the iGABA cells, human GABAergic neurons derived from iPSCs. More precisely, those iGABA cells were mostly cortical GABAergic neurons, which in HD patients start degenerating in the late stages of disease. It would have been relevant including in our *in vitro* experiments human iPSCs-derived MSNs (Golas, 2018), whose loss is considered one of the main hallmarks of HD.

Although scarce reports indicate the presence of mHTT within microglia (Crotti et al., 2014; Maxan et al., 2018), it would have also been interesting to incubate human iPSCs-derived microglia with HTTExon1 fibrils or even generate a coculture of iPSCs-derived microglia and iPSCs-derived MSNs. This coculture would help to demonstrate if the fibrils equally propagate, seed and induce morphological or cell-specific pathological changes in the two lines. Alternatively, the presence of microglia could exert a protective role phagocyting and clearing extracellular mHTT.

• **Technical issues related to the study of mHTT uptake**. According to Ruiz-Arlandis et al., HTTExon1 fibrils are internalized by both differentiated and undifferentiated SH-SY5Y cells via clathrin-dependent endocytosis (Ruiz-Arlandis et al., 2016). In our study, it would have been interesting to verify if the fibrils can be uptaken via the same endocytic pathway by the THP1 derived macrophage cells and iGABA neurons, or if different cell lines uptake the same mHTT species using different processes. Using live-imaging, we observed that THP1 derived macrophages cells were particularly motile and tended to uptake the free-floating mHTT fibrils quickly (within 2-4 hours). Their motility was, from a technical point of view, a disadvantage, because it hindered their imaging as they easily slipped out of focus. The neuronal-like and neuronal cells, instead, were initially firmly attached to the dish, but began to die before we could record mHTT fibril uptake. Resolving such technical limitations would have allowed us to study, more in-depth, mHTT fibrils uptake and consequences.

• **Animal model**. Masnata et al. selected the R6/2 mouse model to study the capacity of mHTT fibrils to spread and seed pathology. This model is known to develop a severe and rapid phenotype that does not allow to investigate longer-term treatment effect. KI mouse models, such as the KI140 and zQ175 mice, may have been a suitable host to detect milder behavioral changes and perform long-term assessments.

•	**Methods of injections**. In the study, WT adult mice received a single injection of mHTT fibrils directly into the cerebral tissue. Three months post-injection, the mHTTExon1 fibrils were no longer detectable and the mice had a mild HD-like phenotype. Performing multiple intracortical injections or the use of an intrathecal pump could have been performed to mimic the extracellular mHTT load normally present in HD organisms. In these conditions, mHTT fibrils could have been more easily detected at end of the experimental timeline. Furthermore, a stable influx of mHTTExon1 fibrils could have possibly accentuated behavioral outcomes.

•	**Methods of tissue preparation**. At the end of the behavioral experiments, all animals were anesthetized and perfused with paraformaldehyde (PFA). PFA perfusion was chosen to perform high-quality immunostaining of the entire brain, from the prefrontal cortex to the cerebellum. This technique allowed us to determine, with a certain degree of accuracy, where the fibrils had spread. However, the use of PFA as a fixation agent comes with a drawback. PFA cross-links the proteins in the tissue, altering the original protein structure and restricting the post-mortem analyses to immunohistochemistry and immunofluorescence. Another animal cohort could have been run in parallel to perform more extensive and diversified post-mortem analyses to investigate mHTTExon1 seeding properties.

2.4 Perspective

Taken together, there is now compelling evidence, with a large part emerging from *in vitro* and more recently from *in vivo* studies (**Table 2 and 5**), that mHTT, as for other proteins linked to neurodegenerative diseases, may behave in a prion-like fashion. However, given that HD is driven by a single gene that leads to the expression of mHTT in every cell of the body, is this of any relevance to the disease burden/onset? And can these propagation mechanisms be used for therapeutic benefits?

Because of the monogenic nature of HD, the relevance of the prion-like behavior of mHTT to the clinic is constantly challenged. Nevertheless, our experimental evidence and published works might indicate that propagating and seeding mHTT species influence HD onset and clinical development in either *in vitro* or *in vivo* systems. For instance, Ast and colleagues identified the presence of mHTT seeding competent species in KI HD mice 10 months prior to symptoms onset, suggesting that these seeds can track disease development (Ast et al., 2018). The same seeds were detected in transgenic models of HD as well as in the caudate nucleus and cerebral cortex of HD patients and correlated with cellular dysfunction and toxicity (Ast et al., 2018).

In light of this evidence, it would be pertinent to identify seeding competent mHTT species in human biological fluids such as the CSF, plasma and saliva. Their concentrations could then be correlated with the subjects' familiar history, HD signs and clinical measures. The group of interest would be mainly composed of pre-symptomatic and early symptomatic patients. CSF mHTT titer is currently used as a biological marker in HD clinical studies (Tabrizi et al., 2019), therefore even given the minimal amount of mHTT in the biological fluids, it could be a feasible procedure to carry out. If mHTT competent seeds are established as a good biomarker of disease, it would further demonstrate the relevance of mHTT extracellular content and of its prion-like capacities in HD. Furthermore, if a correlation with a specific seed is identified, it could explain the discrepancy observed in the clinical trials (e.g. IONIS-HTTRx) between the decrease of unspecific CSF mHTT concentrations and the absence of clinical improvement. The identification of mHTT competent seeds can be then used to template new therapeutic approaches such as the design of antibodies or intrabodies.

Another therapeutic strategy could consist of preventing mHTT spreading. In many disorders, including HD, transsynaptic/transneuronal spreading may be the favored route of protein transfer. Exocytosis, which occurs at the synaptic terminal, is regulated by a number of proteins, some of which interact pre- or post-synaptically with HTT. Consequently, mHTT can interfere with normal synaptic transmission by sequestering the WT protein, a phenomenon that is exacerbated as the polyQ length increases (Smith et al., 2005). The work of Pecho-Vrieseling and colleagues has provided evidence that mHTT itself can circulate between the pre- and post-synaptic membrane. Administration of BoNT - which works by cleaving and inactivating SNARE proteins (SNAP25 and VAMP-2) - blocked exocytosis and consequently mHTT transsynaptic propagation throughout the cortico-striatal pathway (Pecho-Vrieseling et al., 2014).

mTOR inhibitors have demonstrated to successfully rescue cortico-striatal degeneration in organotypic-striatal cultures derived from R6/2 and *Hdh*Q150 HD mouse models. mTOR regulates a wide variety of cell functions - including autophagy downregulation - and the mTOR inhibitor AZD8055 has been shown to decrease the size of mHTT aggregates and the amount of insoluble mHTT in MSNs in both the models cited above (Proenca et al., 2013). mTOR inhibitors have also been found to reduce mHTT accumulation and alleviate toxicity in fly and mouse models of HD (Ravikumar et al., 2004), prevent levo-dopa induced dyskinesias in mouse models of PD (Santini et al., 2009) and ameliorate cognitive deficits in various AD animal models (C. Wang et al., 2014).

Transneuronal propagation of pathological proteins is not a unique characteristic of mHTT. It has been demonstrated for tau and Aβ in AD (de Calignon et al., 2012; Lee et al., 2012; Wu et al., 2013) and α-syn in PD (Angot et al., 2012; Desplats et al., 2009; Freundt et al., 2012; Luk et al., 2012a, 2012b; Rey et al., 2016). Of great relevance is the fact that transneuronal spread of α-syn can be blocked by the monoclonal antibody 1H7 *in vitro* (Games et al., 2014) and *in vivo* (Spencer et al., 2017), ameliorating axonal transport and synaptic trafficking, and raising the possibility of also treating HD through passive immunization. While the release of vesicles containing tau and α-syn is increased by overexpression of the co-chaperone DnaJC5 – possibly through non-canonical SNAP23 exocytosis – this is not the case for mHTT, indicating that not all pathological proteins may behave in the same manner under the same circumstances (Fontaine et al., 2016). We therefore may have to tailor therapies to specifically address the different mechanisms for propagation adopted by each protein, while other treatment options may be applicable to a range of proteins.

Previous reports have also indicated that tunneling nanotubes represent an efficient means for cells to communicate and share material. As we described above, F-actin is the principal component of the nanotube trafficking paths and its depolymerization by latrunculin or by cytochalasin B abolishes the formation of TNTs, or at least reduces the number formed (Bukoreshtliev et al., 2009). If depolymerizing actin may be an attractive target by which to prevent bridge formation between cells – hence mHTT spreading – its implications for microfilaments and microtubules within the cytoskeleton organization would need to be known before applying such methodologies, given the detrimental consequences this may have on the cell integrity. TNT formation is also promoted by oxidative stress, as shown with H_2O_2 administration and serum starvation (Wang et al., 2011). However, interventions designed to control oxidative stress are too non-specific to allow for the generation of a meaningful agent. Additionally, modulations of the M-Sec promoter protein (Hase et al., 2009), tumor suppressor p53, epidermal growth factor receptor (EGFR) and EGFR-regulated Akt, PI3K and mTOR (Wang et al., 2011) could be considered as targets given they all have a direct effect on nanotube growth. Unfortunately, the reduction of physiological levels of any of these transcription factors could have devastating effects on the cell's vital functions.

To prevent the spreading of pathological proteins via TNTs, we could consider targeting the molecules that promote TNT formation. For example, it has been reported that molecular motor myosin-X (Myo10) expression increases the number of TNTs and the transfer of vesicles between co-cultured cells (Gousset et al., 2013). In particular, a specific sequence of Myo10 is required for the formation and function of TNTs (Gousset et al., 2013), and its deletion does not affect filopodia involved in cell-to-cell communication (Bohil et al., 2006). However, it is important to note that TNT formation is beginning to be understood as a process that is cell-specific, in other words, different cell lines can induce TNTs via different mechanisms (Gousset et al., 2013). This is a characteristic that is extremely important to take into consideration if we aim to inhibit TNT production in a specific cell population.

Endocytosis is also a very efficient pathway for mHTT internalization (Ruiz-Arlandis et al., 2016) and therefore could be considered to halt propagation and disease dissemination. For example, chlorpromazine, monodansylcadaverine and dynasore can suppress mHTT uptake in N2A cells by a clathrin-dependent endocytosis mechanism (Ruiz-Arlandis et al., 2016). Although chlorpromazine has been used to treat psychotic disorders since the fifties, it is known to induce side-effects which include tardive dyskinesia, dystonia, motor restlessness and akathisia, which limits its use in a debilitating movement-disorder such as HD. Other pharmacological approaches could be employed to specifically inhibit clathrin-dependent endocytosis but a complete screening should be undertaken to identify such compounds, test their efficacy and monitor their potential side-effects as blocking this pathway could affect the well-being of the cells/neurons and only partially prevent mHTT propagation.

However, blocking mHTT uptake without targeting its release would not provide a fully efficient therapy. In order to address this issue, neutral sphingomyelinase and PI3-kinase inhibitors have been investigated. These compounds have shown the capacity to reduce the secretion of (i) 72Q in transfected N2A cells, (ii) full-length mHTT in rat primary cortical neurons and (iii) endogenous mHTT of HdhQ111/Hdh$^+$ and HdhQ111/HdhQ111 murine striatal cells (Trajkovic et al., 2017). Surprisingly, the knockdown of mHTT secretion by neutral sphingomyelinase inhibitors did not increase the amount of mHTT in the intracellular compartment, neither did it induce cell toxicity, raising the possibility to target release and propagation of free forms of mHTT. Side-effects of PI3-kinase inhibitors were not reported (Trajkovic et al., 2017). The fact that mHTT is very often detected outside the cell boundary, notably in the CSF (Tan et al., 2015; Wild et al., 2015), within the extracellular matrix (Cicchetti et al., 2014), in blood vessels (Drouin-Ouellet et al., 2015) and in plasma (Rieux et al., 2020) may indicate the existence of other release mechanisms. mHTT found in the extracellular milieu is also likely to emerge from cell death driven by mHTT toxicity (Cicchetti et al., 2014).

The plasma membrane constitutes a major barrier to external toxins. To preserve the homeostasis, it is quite selective in determining which compounds can cross or bind to its surface. Interactions between proteins and cell membranes can be physical, such as by electrostatic attractions, or chemical, through specific or non-specific lipid, protein or carbohydrate bindings. In particular, binding of the HTT-N-terminus with the lipids of biological membrane has been shown to be dependent on electrostatic interactions (Kegel et al., 2005). mHTT carries variable repetitions of polyglutamine residues at the N-terminus, and increasing the number of polyQ provides more insertion sites into the lipid bilayer. This occurs via vesicles that simulate the biological membrane, corrupting its integrity (Kegel et al., 2009). Several other studies have demonstrated plasma membrane structural modifications following interactions with tau, Aβ or α-syn (Flach et al., 2012; Zhu et al., 2003). These interactions are well described in studies which compared the properties of α-syn and mHTT fibrils. They have revealed that soluble α-syn fibrils have different binding capacities depending on their charge, while HTTExon1Q41 does not express this specificity, at least as demonstrated in synthetic vesicles (Pieri et al., 2012). It was also shown that HTTExon1 binding is dependent on the number of interaction sites, which is not the case for α-syn (Monsellier et al., 2016). Despite some dissimilarities, α-syn and mHTT fibrils do share common properties such as being able to modify the permeability of the lipid membrane by Ca^{2+} influxes (Monsellier et al., 2016). Furthermore, cholesterol concentration in the phospholipid bilayer impacts on its rigidity and stability, challenging the fibrils' capacity to alter the membrane's permeability (Pieri et al., 2012). In this regard, ethyl-EPA dampened motor deficits in an HD mouse model (Clifford et al., 2002), probably due to its property to positively influence the plasma membrane properties, by preventing oxidative stress (Puri et al., 2005) or inhibiting apoptotic pathways (Murck and Manku, 2007). Unfortunately, even if this compound has already completed a phase III clinical trial with some evidence of efficacy (Puri et al., 2005), subsequent investigations failed to reach the primary outcome measures (Ferreira et al., 2015)

It is becoming clear that mHTT propagation is associated with significant pathological changes. Although it is of importance to understand how mHTT spreads, accesses the cellular compartment and eventually recruits HTT, targeting the mechanisms of mHTT propagation may not be the most efficient therapeutic strategy. For instance, inhibiting a single mHTT propagation pathway could be ineffective, while addressing all of them could be potentially detrimental to cellular homeostasis. In fact, synaptic transmission, TNTs formation, exocytosis, endocytosis and plasma membrane integrity are fundamental cellular functions that need to be preserved.

As of now, disease-modifying treatments for HD are not available, but several approaches aiming at reducing mHTT levels are currently developed and tested. Lowering mHTT can be achieved by promoting mHTT degradation or preventing its synthesis. In homeostatic conditions, mHTT is degraded by macroautophagy and the ubiquitin-proteasome system. While simply enhancing the activity of these systems might disrupt cellular equilibrium, autophagosome-tethering compounds as well as proteolysis-targeting chimeras have been designed to boost mHTT-specific clearance via these systems (Li et al., 2019; Sakamoto et al., 2001).

Gene silencing approaches aim instead to lower mHTT by inhibiting its synthesis. Different gene silencing therapies are currently being tested in clinical trials and are yielding some positive outcomes. However, technical disadvantages (i.e. invasive mode of delivery and poor pharmacokinetics properties) and uncertainties (i.e. side effects of unspecifically targeting *HTT*, overall efficacy, and identification of ideal candidates for the treatment) are related to the application of these methodologies.

One of the most important concerns relates to the issue of non-selectively when targeting the mutated allele. So far, lowering both HTT and mHTT synthesis via ASO (IONIS-HTTRx) or microRNA (AMT-130) did not cause any major side-effects (Caron et al., 2020; Tabrizi et al., 2019). However, convincing evidence is pointing out that HTT is essential for the maintenance of functional synaptic connectivity and for striatal cell survival (Burrus et al., 2020; McAdam et al., 2020; Poplawski et al., 2020) and, as such, its expression has to be preserved. Furthermore, in case of non-selective allele silencing approach, it is important to consider that while ASOs therapy temporally blocks protein synthesis, viral transductions with microRNAs or CRISPRCas9 could permanently halt the target-protein transcription. Thus, inhibiting the synthesis of mHTT alone, as ASO drugs WVE-120101 and WVE-120102 do (Wave Life Sciences Ltd., 2020a, 2020b), could be a safer strategy.

HTT gene silencing treatments successfully decreased mHTT CSF titer without significant side effects, but, so far, failed to improve motor or cognitive symptoms (Tabrizi et al., 2019; Wave Life Sciences Ltd., 2020a, 2020b). The cause of these outcomes is still unknown. A low drug dosage could be one of the reasons (Wave Life Sciences Ltd., 2020a, 2020b). However, considering that progressive accumulation of mHTT in the CNS is one of the main pathological hallmarks of HD, downregulating *HTT* translation could not be sufficient to compensate for the amount of mHTT already present in the system at the time of the treatment. It would be, therefore, advantageous to start HTT lowering therapies as early as possible (pre-manifest or early stage). In this scenario, genetic testing and the use of accurate biomarkers would be fundamental to select optimal candidates for these treatments.

HD being a genetic disorder, silencing or editing the mutated gene could generate efficient anti-HD treatments. However, in manifest patients, this therapeutic intervention could be insufficient to treat the disease because it does not address the extensive load of intracellular and extracellular mHTT already present in the CNS and in the periphery. To consider this aspect of the pathology, combinational therapy could be adopted to target intracellular mHTT by inhibiting its synthesis (gene silencing/editing) or promoting its clearance (intrabody), as well as to block extracellular mHTT propagation (antibody therapy) (**Figure 2.1**). Antibody therapy via active or passive immunization could be useful and would not interfere with the primary aim of gene silencing/editing methodologies. Furthermore, anti-mHTT antibody treatments could block mHTT propagation and consequent seeding without disturbing main biological functions.

Future therapeutic perspectives will need to converge and tackle this genetic disorder from several fronts, including both pre-manifest and manifest patients, using combinations of agents that inhibit mHTT synthesis; restrict the damaging effects of the protein portion that is then secreted and by so doing prevent the accumulation and spread of this pathogenic protein (**Figure 2.1**).

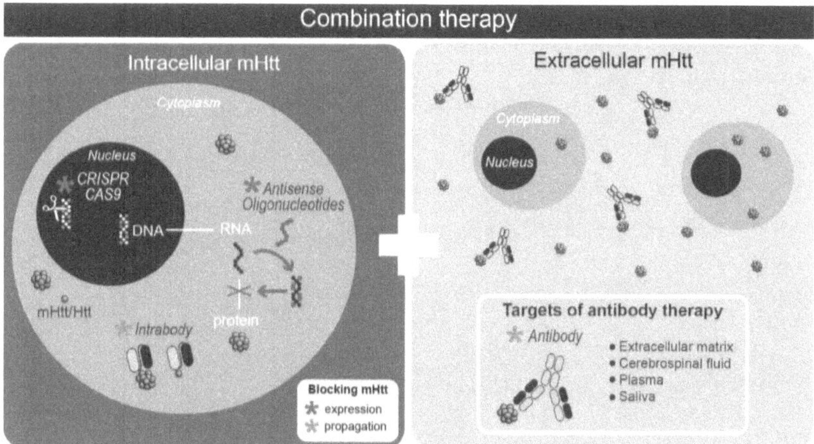

Figure 2.1. Target intracellular and extracellular mHTT via combination therapy. The inhibition of mHTT expression (gene silencing/editing) and propagation (antibody treatment) could represent the future of combinational therapy to successfully target both intracellular and extracellular mHTT. Abbreviations: CAS9, CRISPR associated protein 9; CRISPR, clustered regularly interspaced short palindromic repeats; DNA, deoxyribonucleic acid; mHTT, mutant huntingtin; mRNA, messenger ribonucleic acid; RNA, ribonucleic acid. Sources (Denis et al., 2019).